# UROGENITAL MANIPULATION

# Urogenital Manipulation

Jean-Pierre Barral

ILLUSTRATIONS BY
Jacques Roth

Eastland Press
SEATTLE

Originally published as *Manipulations uro-génitales,* Maloine (Paris), 1987, with additional material drawn from *Nouvelles techniques uro-génitales,* Maloine (Paris), 1992.

English language edition © 1993, 2006 by Eastland Press, Inc.
P.O. Box 99749
Seattle, WA 98139, USA
*www.eastlandpress.com*

Library of Congress Catalog Card Number: 93-72643
International Standard Book Number. 0-939616-18-1
Printed in the United States of America

English language edition edited by
Stephen Anderson, Ph.D. & Daniel Bensky, D.O.

6 8 10 9 7 5

Book design by Gary Niemeier

"Tell the boys to keep it Pure. Tell the boys to keep it Pure."

—*Final advice of A.T. Still spoken to W.C. Dawes, D.O.*

# Table of Contents

# *Foreword*

I am honored to write the foreword for this book. I feel very strongly about the importance of this series on visceral manipulation by Dr. Barral. These books are so significant because they focus on a considerable void in traditional Western health care today, i.e., working directly with the organs and their adjacent and supportive tissues to restore their normal structure/function and motion relationships. This helps unleash their potential for health. Conventional Western medical training includes surgical and pharmacologic approaches to organ dysfunctions. Osteopathic training adds manipulation of the musculoskeletal system to affect the various organ systems through the nervous and circulatory systems. Until now, however, osteopathic literature has only included brief and unsystematic mentions of directly manipulating the organs.

On the one hand, the approach taken in this book is reductionistic in its precise focus on anatomic and diagnostic specificity. It is also integrative (or wholistic) in its awareness of the impact of specific dysfunctions on every aspect of the person. In this way it demonstrates how the two approaches can coexist synergistically and lead to a higher order of patient care.

The functional anatomy of the pelvis is explained clearly and concisely. The principles of diagnosis and treatment techniques are described in such a way that they can be grasped easily and applied experientially. Clinical and philosophical pearls are contained throughout and communicated in a gentle, benevolent style. Still, their application will require a significant amount of study and practice. These techniques are precise and subtle, yet very powerful in mobilizing the body's own healing capabilities.

The presentation is clear and intellectually honest, which makes it both palatable and accessible. The descriptions of anatomy, physiology, and pathophysiology are carefully detailed so that the reader can be confident in applying the work in the clinic. The presentation facilitates a rational understanding of how the diagnostics and treatments can work using a structure/function perspective. The diagnostic tests and treatments have been validated with laboratory and imaging studies, as well as clinical experience with a large number of patients. The contraindications section is well thought-out and explained. It demonstrates an understanding of the practitioner's role in the complex environment of contemporary health care, and not from the cure-all point of view of an isolationist.

As osteopathic physicians, we have an obligation to restore normal functioning of the various systems of the human body using manipulation. Our training has emphasized the regulation of the body through the nervous and circulatory systems. This book, and the series as a whole, takes manipulation a step further by working directly on the organs and their surrounding tissues. This helps restore the normal structure/function relationships which cannot be addressed pharmacologically or via neuromusculoskeletal relationships. The diagnostic and treatment techniques in this book are essential to the complete care of patients with urogenital problems. They are equal in importance to pharmacologic and surgical approaches, and should be used in conjunction with them.

I have been the coordinator of Osteopathic Manipulative Medicine (OMM) at one of the 15 osteopathic colleges in the United States for the past 13 years. It is exciting to contemplate integrating the information presented in this book into our OMM curriculum. Even more exciting is the idea of integrating it into our Basic Science and Physician Skills/Physical Diagnosis courses. This will enable our graduates to more completely evaluate and treat dysfunctions of the organ systems. The other area which this book (and the whole series) can stimulate is clinical research. This is sorely needed in order for our profession to demonstrate its efficacy, and to help make this modality more a part of mainstream health care.

Dr. Still told us that life is motion. Dr. Barral tells us that osteopathy is the study of motion. In this book he takes us on a most precise and refined exploration of the motions of the urogenital system, enabling us to develop a detailed understanding of the structures and their functional relationships. We can also better understand the forces acting on them and within them. He shares with us how we can use our hands to interact with these organs and tissues. This interaction helps the body to restore more ideal motion and thereby improve their function. In this way we can successfully treat many of the problems in the urogenital area which otherwise plague some people's lives.

When I was in osteopathic medical school we were taught one of Dr. Still's metaphors. He said that osteopathy was like mining a very pure grade of ore, and that D.O. stood for "Dig On." We were told to continue mining this seam of ore to further expose the elegance and power of this natural approach to working with patients. The goal was that people could experience their full potential for health. Dr. Sutherland was held up as an example for us to follow. He selflessly dedicated his life to "unearthing" osteopathy as it applies to the cranium and the central nervous system. Both of these men stayed true to the essence of this "seam of ore" called osteopathy. As we read and experience this, the fourth book in his series on visceral manipulation, we find that Dr. Barral too is staying true to this pure seam of ore in all its elegance and power.

At a time when we are at a loss to define the distinctiveness of osteopathy, reading this book will put us back "in touch" with it. In addition, it will rekindle our enthusiasm to practice osteopathy.

Tom Shaver, D.O
Lewisburg, WV

# Chapter One:
## Introduction

# Table of Contents

# *Introduction*

In our earlier book *Visceral Manipulation* (English version published in 1988), my colleague Pierre Mercier and I were only able to briefly introduce the topic of urogenital manipulation. *Visceral Manipulation* was, of course, a general introductory textbook, and we had to cover many different organ systems. The present book is devoted solely to urogenital manipulation.

Although written by one person, this book will use the first person plural voice. A person in our field who "places himself upon an island" is committing the sin of pride. How can one overlook those instructors and colleagues who provide the background and support system of our osteopathic culture? Whatever knowledge and skill we may have today is due largely to their help and teaching.

We became interested in urogenital manipulation very early in our practice because of the numerous urogenital problems we encountered. Many of our female patients complained of such problems as dyspareunia and especially urinary incontinence. They felt abandoned by conventional medicine and considered the results of surgery inadequate.

We view the human body as an organic, functional entity. We were puzzled by the fact that the urogenital system often seems to be viewed differently from other body systems (i.e., largely ignored) by medical practitioners and patients alike. One obvious reason for this is culturally programmed "modesty." The early anatomical texts were written by monks. How did they refer to the urogenital system? As the *pudendalis* system, i.e., the system to be ashamed of! This stigma remained even as medicine became secularized. Many physicians assumed the role of defenders of morality, and their attitude toward parts of the body having sexual or excretory functions was shaped by prevailing social taboos and inhibitions as much as by practical medical considerations.

Concerned by our patients' problems, we gradually discovered ways to therapeutically manipulate the urogenital area. From the outset, we were impressed both by the subtlety required for these techniques and by their effectiveness. It was interesting to compare the enthusiasm of our patients with the disinterest of conventional medical practitioners. Thanks to the continued positive feedback from our patients, our understanding and abilities in this area have evolved and improved.

At first, even our osteopathic colleagues were guarded in their opinions about our work with the urogenital system. Some of them were in total disagreement with our efforts. Now, fifteen years later, it is interesting to note that in Europe (especially France) the student who wishes to pass the final exams in osteopathy must usually demonstrate competence in urogenital manipulation.

The true beneficiaries of these techniques are the women who take advantage of them to feel better and, in some cases, avoid surgery. To us, it makes no sense for a practitioner of manual medicine to deliberately avoid the urogenital area. Considered simply from a biomechanical perspective, these tissues are among the most stressed in the body because of the effects of pregnancy, delivery, menstruation, lumbosacral dysfunction, intestinal problems, lower limb restrictions, psychological/emotional phenomena, etc. As health professionals, we have an obligation to help our patients in whatever way is appropriate.

Although we naturally used standard anatomical, physiological, and medical texts as sources, most of the material presented here is derived from our own clinical experience, using our own hands. Our knowledge is derived from countless osteopathic consultations, and most of the techniques described have been used thousands of times. We present only the techniques that have been clinically or experimentally verified as being useful. For this purpose, we have used various imaging technologies including ultrasound and fluoroscopy. We prefer the latter because it enables one to follow and modify the movement of an organ in its normal planes of motion.

Aware of the impact a book can have, we have limited descriptions and discussions to those things that we have seen in the normal course of our practice. When in doubt about some point of anatomy or aspect of treatment, we prefer to refrain from making any comments. It is our belief that our profession already suffers too much from uncertainties and theories that are both imaginative and illusionary.

It is a fact that osteopathy is an empirical form of medicine. It is quite difficult to prove that a hand can have an effect on the human frame. Proving it repeatedly is that much more difficult. To state that osteopathy is a science would be to ignore the craft of the practitioner and, more importantly, the concept that every patient is unique. Perhaps the reality is that conventional medicine is not much more "scientific" in this regard.

The information which is given by our hands must be received, integrated, and activated by the patient's body. Demonstrating the local effect of our manipulations is not at all the same as proving that manipulation can have a general effect within the body. This general effect depends not only on the patient's physical organism but also on their education, general culture, and personality. These are issues that are struggled with by all health practitioners.

It is vitally important that we continue to deal with the mainstream medical world and its technological prowess. Any group which is too insular and self-absorbed can only too quickly drift towards unreasonable ideas and techniques.

# *General*

## VERTEBRAL COLUMN AND SKULL

Although our primary subject here is manipulation of the urogenital system, we must caution the reader against reductionism. It is the osteopath's responsibility to test and treat all articulations. Stillian osteopathy is essentially a vertebral osteopathy. Even the best visceral techniques, without the support of vertebral correction, will not give optimal results. The classic text by Irvin Korr on this subject (1978), which covers the neurobiological mechanisms of vertebral restrictions and their sequelae, is recommended reading.

In a patient who presents with an L1/L2 restriction, for example, all tissues in the corresponding dermatomes are likely to have abnormal tonus. This affects arterial, venous, and lymphatic circulation in such a way that any trauma, pathogenic agent, or decompensating factor is able to provoke a restriction out of proportion to the cause.

The above reasoning works both ways. Following untreated vertebral restrictions, or after a direct trauma (such as surgery) or infection, it is important that the viscera be manipulated. An untreated visceral restriction can gradually lead to a vertebral restriction which, in a "vicious circle," further aggravates the visceral problem. Osteopathy is a holistic form of medicine, and we urge our readers to shun the reductionist point of view.

## MOBILITY AND MOTILITY

In *Visceral Manipulation* (pp. 5-12) we discussed the different movements of the organism according to the system which influences or controls them:

- somatic nervous system
- autonomic nervous system
- craniosacral system (also known as primary respiratory motion)
- visceral motility.

Below we will review and expand on these topics, focusing on those aspects which were insufficiently explained or in which our knowledge has increased. If the reader has not already read *Visceral Manipulation*, we remind him to do so before continuing with this book.

### Mobility

This is the passive or active visible motion of a structure. The motion is in response either to the somatic nervous system (gross physical movement) or to the motion of the diaphragm during breathing. Osteopathy is the art of diagnosing a loss of mobility within the body and bringing about a correction. We have had to repeatedly argue for this concept of mobility. Some people believe that osteopathy accomplishes nothing because x-rays taken before and after treatment often document no change. But what do photographs (or x-rays for that matter) of an automobile engine before and after repair show?

From the osteopathic viewpoint it matters very little if a particular articulation, organ, or cranial bone is deformed or in an asymmetrical position. What matters is whether it is mobile. A retroverted and fixed uterus is pathogenic; a retroverted but mobile uterus is fully functional. A fixed scoliosis is pathogenic; a mobile scoliosis is functional, and so on. This view of structure and function is one of osteopathy's great strengths.

New theories and approaches in osteopathy come and go, but none has ever denied the importance of structure. A. T. Still, the great pioneer in the field, stated unequivocally that structure governs function. We have consistently found this to be true. When a structure can no longer be mobilized, when fibrous tissues replace elastic tissues, when arteries, nerves, or lymphatic systems are trapped in a stranglehold—then illness appears.

Still's statement that "the rule of the artery is supreme" did not, of course, imply that direct manipulation of an artery is our goal in treatment, rather that it is of the utmost importance to free the structural environment of the artery. Likewise, osteopathy is not about bone diseases and an osteopath is not a bonesetter; rather an osteopath is a manipulator of the soft tissues which surround the bones or insert into them.

It is very difficult to localize and distinguish between the various palpated and tested tissues in the pelvic area. Only by having a *thorough knowledge* of both external and internal anatomy can we accomplish this. When we test mobility, we are looking for tissues which have abnormal elasticity, distensibility, or sensitivity. Our tests and perceptions must be extremely delicate and precise, given the delicacy of the organs and tissues we are treating.

## Motility

In contrast to mobility (the visible extrinsic movement of a structure in response to its environment), motility is the innate, *intrinsic* motion of a structure, occurring independently of the causes of mobility. Many viscera possess an intrinsic motion of low frequency (approximately 7 cycles per minute) and low amplitude, generally invisible to the naked eye.

The ability to reliably and reproducibly detect motility demands considerable (typically many years) experience in palpation. Several accomplished practitioners, their hands upon the same subject, can perceive the same motility and detect, simultaneously and immediately, an artificially-induced perturbation of the motility. We have performed experiments of this type dozens of times, taking all possible precautions to ensure objectivity. The results were quite clear and convincing to us. Yet, use of medical technology has so far been unable to confirm our perceptions of motility. This remains a great dilemma. Is the human hand capable of detecting something which a machine cannot? We have had high hopes for magnetic nuclear resonance, but some of the functional limitations of this imaging technology have so far prevented it from being helpful in this regard.

Some osteopaths have suggested that motility is an effect of "primary respiratory motion" (i.e., fluctuation of cerebrospinal fluid). We believe it is more accurately considered to be the result of cellular "memory" of embryological movements, which are reproduced in motility. In other words, the motion which occurs during motility represents an oscillation between accentuation of the embryological movement and a return to the original position. In order to differentiate those movements which are due to movements of the diaphragm, we use the terms "expir" and "inspir" (*Visceral Manipulation*, pp. 8-12). Expir moves a given organ closer to the median axis, whereas inspir moves it away (*Illustration 1-1*). In the case of organs located on the median axis, inspir moves them anteriorly while expir moves them posteriorly.

Tests of motility are also known as motility listening techniques. Techniques for normalizing motility are usually called "induction," which combines listening and direct action. You start out by listening to and following the motility. Once you know which half of the cycle has a larger amplitude and vitality, you accentuate that half and merely follow the other half, and continue this until you feel that the whole motility cycle has become easy and free (see *Visceral Manipulation*, pp. 23-24).

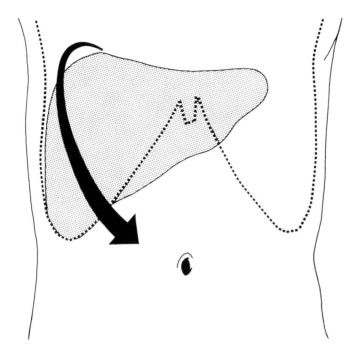

**Illustration 1-1**
Motility of Liver (Expir)

## LISTENING

We should clarify our use of the term "listening." According to our concept, you place your hand lightly on an area and passively concentrate on the motion of the tissues. It is important to distinguish this technique from types of palpation in which you extend your sense of touch (e.g., feeling for motility or primary respiration). In listening, you "attract" the body toward your hand instead of actively extending your sense of touch away from your hand through the body. With practice, your hand will be drawn to the most important restricted area. For more information, see *Visceral Manipulation II* (1989), pp. 8-12.

### General Listening

When listening to the head of a standing or seated subject, you obtain information about the whole body. This is called general listening, and is typically performed at the beginning of a session to determine the general location of a restriction. In the seated position, the subject's legs should be slightly apart. Stand behind, place one hand on the posterior skull and the other under the sacrum, and let the body express itself *(Illustration 1-2)*. You will get a sense of the laterality and level of a restriction:

- the body will sidebend toward the affected side
- the greater the sidebending, the lower down in the body is the restriction.

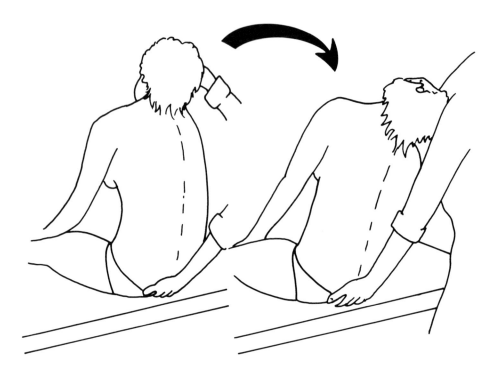

**Illustration 1-2**
General Listening

If the most important restriction is in one of the lower limbs, you may feel nothing (because the seated position makes feeling past the pelvis too difficult), or the sidebending may be so great that the head touches the table. Forward and backward bending also reflect the level of restriction, especially for midline problems. For example, with a vertebral column restriction, the back of the neck tends to move closer to the sacrum. A large anteroposterior movement usually indicates a coccygeal restriction. These signs are clearest with the subject in the standing position.

## Local Listening

Local listening is performed on a specific area such as the thorax or lower abdomen, and enables you to determine the exact location of a restriction. For the lower abdomen, place the heel of your more sensitive hand over the pubic symphysis, with the middle finger on the midline pointing to the umbilicus. The movement of the palm (not that of the fingers) indicates the direction of the urogenital problem. When the restriction has been precisely localized, the heel of the hand stops moving and becomes pronated or supinated. At the end, only the pisiform or the first metacarpophalangeal joint is in contact with the body.

Effective osteopathic technique requires extreme manual delicacy and sensitivity. Our hands, placed on any part of the body, are attracted to abnormal tissue tension, which may be of muscular, fascial, neurovascular, articular, or visceral origin. When the hand comes into contact with the affected zone, the attraction which was drawing it stops.

In visceral manipulation, local listening is indispensable. It frequently shows us the area requiring treatment when neither palpation, nor mobility testing, nor questioning are sufficient. The body knows where its own problems lie, and draws the practitioner's hand to that area.

In both France and America, we have frequently accepted "challenges," in which we are asked to manually diagnose restrictions which have been previously documented by other means. Our record of success in these challenges is quite good.

In one variation, after your hand has been drawn to a particular organ (e.g., the liver), you continue local listening with your hand positioned directly over the organ. Your hand may then go in a certain direction following a line of tension corresponding to expir or inspir; this tells you whether the organ is in relative expir or inspir. If you feel nothing, the organ may either be normal or "frozen." A frozen organ is one in which the motility is of such a low amplitude that it cannot be palpated. Local listening cannot differentiate the normal from the frozen; for that you must check the motility.

Local listening using the external abdominal/pelvic approach is described below. Internal techniques (described later) also utilize this sensation of the tissues pulling our hand, which enhances their precision. Common findings for various organs are shown in *Illustration 1-3*.

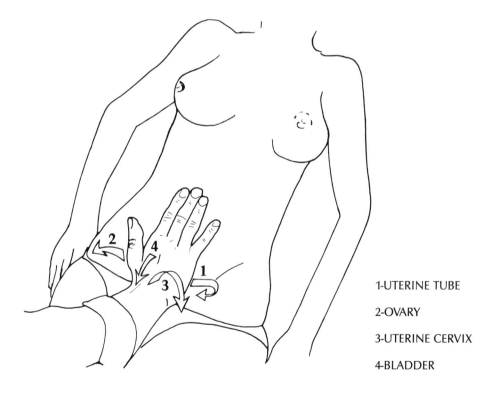

**Illustration 1-3**
Local Listening: Pelvis

1-UTERINE TUBE

2-OVARY

3-UTERINE CERVIX

4-BLADDER

UTERINE TUBE: The palm of the hand slides slightly laterally (~1 cm), then either pronates (for a restriction of the right tube) or supinates (left tube) (see arrow #1). While rotating, the palm almost imperceptibly pushes inward posteriorly. This impression is more noticeable when the uterine cervix is involved. With tubal restrictions, the palm tends to be drawn toward the uterotubal junction. This may also happen following infection or miscarriage. The passage of time does not diminish the phenomena of local listening. Even if our own minds forget, the body never does!

OVARY: The palm slides farther laterally than for the uterine tubes, and stops at a point approximately at the junction of a parasagittal line and a transverse line passing through the anterosuperior iliac spines (A.S.I.S.) and the pubic symphysis respectively. The palm then pushes posteriorly very slightly (see arrow #2). There is often a slight rotation over the affected ovary. We have encountered more tubal problems than ovarian problems. This may be due in part to the high incidence of pelvic inflammatory disease.

UTERINE CERVIX: You immediately feel a distinct supination or pronation of the heel of the hand, and the palm pushes deep posteriorly (see arrow #3).

BLADDER: Local listening for the bladder is difficult to differentiate from that for the uterine cervix. However, for the bladder the motion is almost always directed posteriorly toward the sacrum on the midline, without rotation in the transverse plane (see arrow #4), and the magnitude of the posterior motion is less than for the cervix.

Of course, your hand may be attracted by other structures during local listening for the pelvis. If there is a small intestine restriction, the heel will move superiorly and then posteriorly. With a sigmoid colon restriction, the heel will move left and then posteriorly without any rotation.

## IMPORTANT TESTS

### Genitohumeral Test

The name of this test may seem incongruous. It reflects a functional correlation between the genital system and the area of the shoulder joint. The test should be performed whenever you encounter periarthritis of the shoulder, cervicobrachial neuralgia, or any inexplicable restriction of shoulder movement in combination with a suspected genital problem. This situation is most common shortly before or after menopause, or in women with prior urogenital problems.

EXTERNAL APPROACH: This test takes advantage of the fact that most shoulder pain worsens with the arm in external abduction/rotation ("candlestick position"). The patient should be supine, with the suspected arm in candlestick position (or, if pain becomes excessive, the beginning of candlestick position).

For the right arm, use your left hand to gradually move the patient's right hand until reaching the limit of mobility allowed by the pain. With your right hand, carry out pressure/inhibition (in the direction of listening) at the pelvic zone revealed by local listening (Illustration 1-4). If there is a connection between the genital system and the shoulder (in most cases ipsilateral), you will feel an immediate improvement in shoulder mobility. This is very similar to the glenohumeral articulation test in which we inhibit hepatic or renal zones of restriction (Visceral Manipulation II, p. 19).

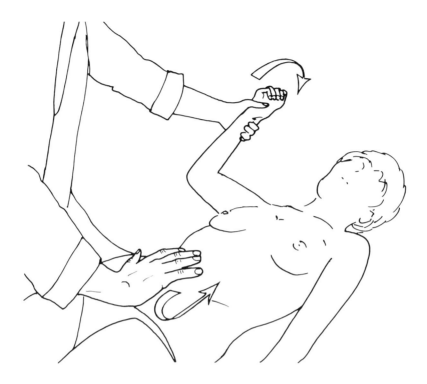

**Illustration 1-4**
Genitohumeral Test: External Approach

INTERNAL APPROACH: This test can be done by replacing the abdominal hand by one or two fingers in the vagina. Again, the fingers move in the direction indicated by listening to inhibit the restriction. This test requires considerable expertise. We advise beginners to start with the external approach.

## Hip Articulation Test

This is analogous to the shoulder technique described above. For cases of hip or upper thigh pain not attributable to an articular problem, carry out pressure/inhibition on the restricted zone of the ipsilateral pelvis. If there is a connection with the genital system, this treatment will produce a noticeable improvement in hip mobility.

## Completed Lasègue Test

This test is appropriate in cases of sciatica with suspected genital system involvement.

BY INHIBITION: With the patient supine, use one hand to lift the leg until movement is limited by pain. Then, use your other hand to perform external pressure/inhibition on the pelvic zone previously indicated by local listening or other means *(Illustration*

1-5). If there is a genital system problem associated with the sciatica, mobility of the leg may be increased by up to 30%.

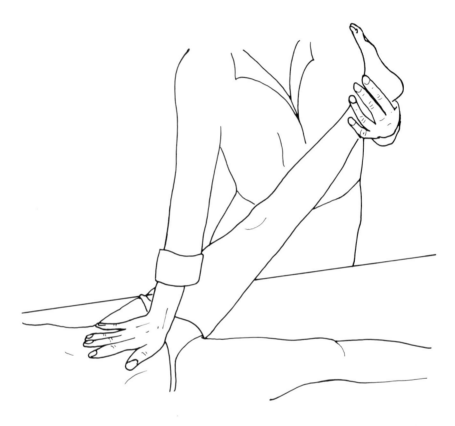

**Illustration 1-5**
Completed Lasègue Test

BY AGGRAVATION: In the same position, lift the leg but stop before the onset of pain. Instead of performing pressure/inhibition, press down on the indicated pelvic zone fairly hard in order to aggravate it. This should be done in the direction opposite to local listening, pressing harder and exaggerating the movement. If there is genital system involvement, this treatment (without moving the leg) will induce pain in the areas supplied by the sciatic nerve (positive result of completed Lasègue test).

## EVALUATION OF OUR TECHNIQUES

Dissection, ultrasound, and fluoroscopy have been useful to us in evaluating our techniques. We would like to thank Professor Arnaud and the late Dr. Roulet for making the dissections possible, and the imaging specialists Drs. Cohen, Constantin, and Behr for enthusiastically making available their equipment and expertise in ultrasound and fluoroscopy. With the help of these specialists, we have been able to compare various techniques and retain only the most effective. Interestingly, only fluoroscopy clearly revealed the effects of urogenital manipulation. It is unfortunate that this imaging mode poses a health risk to the researcher and therefore cannot be used extensively. These three evaluation methods enabled us to confirm:

- the accuracy of manual diagnosis;
- the ability of the hand to effect change;
- the predominance of mobility over position.

In one patient, using mobility tests, we discovered a right obturator bladder restriction. This was documented by fluoroscopy when, with each movement of forced exhalation, the fixed side of the bladder collapsed. We have also used fluoroscopy to check our ability to release restrictions and restore physiologic motion to the bladder. Seeing

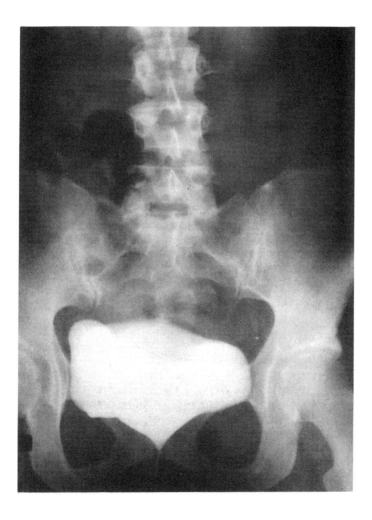

**Illustration 1-6**
Cystography: Right Obturator Foramen Restriction

one's hands locate and release a restriction is a useful and reassuring form of "positive feedback" for the therapist.

In general, radiography simply shows a structure at a certain moment in time and therefore gives information on position but not physiology. This was illustrated in our study of a patient with bladder ptosis and associated urinary incontinence during strenuous activity. Upon examination, we found a restriction in the right obturator foramen. We performed cystography, which showed that the right side of the bladder was a little lower than the left and went slightly past the upper border of the obturator foramen *(Illustration 1-6)*. This restriction, which produced the incontinence, was not visible with simple radiography. It is interesting to note that our hands found this first. In fact, the average radiologist would probably have noticed nothing abnormal about the image. After we released the restriction, the incontinence disappeared but there was no observable change on cystography. Only the dynamics had changed; the static relationship between the organ and its environment remained the same. After treatment, the bladder was able to move harmoniously with the structures that surrounded it, i.e., it was not the position but the original restriction which was pathogenic. This is a good example of the difference between osteopathic and conventional approaches.

Using imaging technology, we were able to see exactly how various techniques affected the mobility of specific structures. Results were not always what we expected. This evaluation allowed us to improve some of our techniques and eliminate others. We demonstrated that induction techniques had a significant effect upon the uterus and its attachments which, as we shall see, all have contractile muscular fibers. Using fluoroscopy, we observed a retroverted uterus correct itself by approximately $30^0$ under induction. This change was only temporary, but was nonetheless a striking demonstration of the ability of a hand placed externally on the pelvis to mobilize an organ.

# *Visceral Articulations*

During each active or passive movement, the pelvic viscera slide on one another in predetermined directions. To understand these movements, we need to understand the various types of sliding surfaces and means of connection.

## SLIDING SURFACES

The sliding ability of the viscera requires a minute quantity of serous fluid between the visceral serous membrane and the surrounding structures. The pelvic cavity is extraperitoneal, but has important relationships superiorly with the peritoneum and inferiorly with the subperitoneal pelvic space.

The **peritoneum** covers the bladder and forms a uterovesical pouch between the uterus and bladder. It covers the uterus and passes posteroinferiorly to form a rectouterine pouch ("Douglas's pouch") between the rectum and uterus *(Illustration 1-7)*. The peritoneum connects the pelvic organs to the small intestine, large intestine, and greater omentum. For this reason, a blow to the peritoneum has numerous and complex effects on pelvic stasis and dynamics.

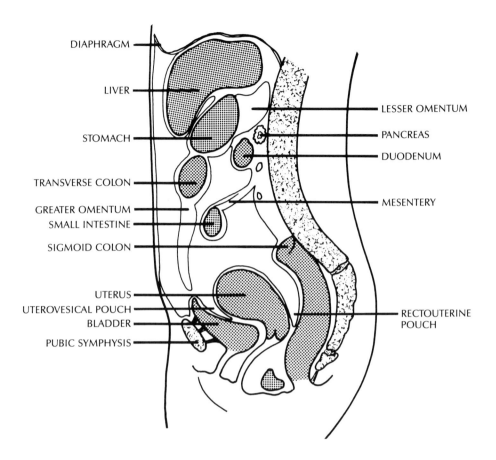

**Illustration 1-7**
Peritoneum with Abdominal and Pelvic Organs

The **subperitoneal pelvic space** fills the space between the peritoneum and the bony/muscular walls of the pelvis. It communicates with the gluteal and obturator regions via the sciatic notch and obturator foramen. It is partitioned by several structures:

- two sagittal peritoneal folds running from the sacrum to the pubis (termed the rectouterine and sacrogenital folds);
- the uterosacral ligaments (reinforced parts of the rectouterine folds);
- the broad ligaments;
- the umbilicoprevesical aponeurosis.

The space contains several important pelvic arteries (internal iliac, uterine, hemorrhoidal, umbilical). There are many smooth muscular fibers which surround the vessels and help support the pelvic organs.

The **perineum** is a group of muscles and associated soft tissues forming the lateral and inferior walls of the pelvis *(Illustrations 1-8 and 1-9)*. It includes:

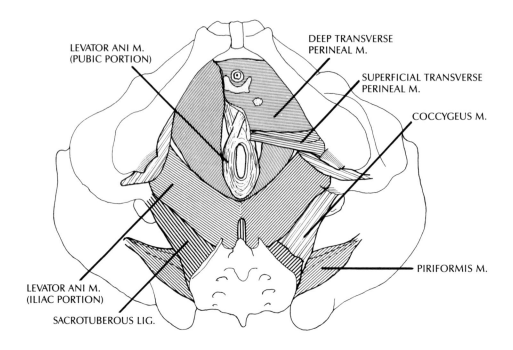

**Illustration 1-8**
Female Perineum: Deep Muscles

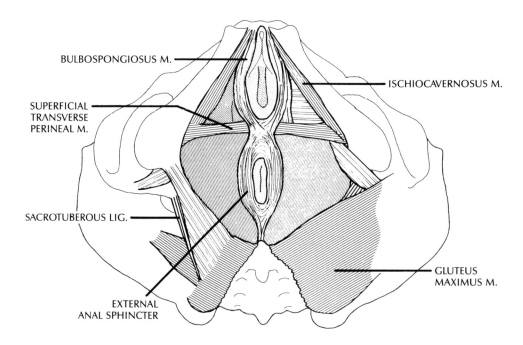

**Illustration 1-9**
Female Perineum: Superficial Muscles

- laterally, the obturator and piriformis muscles and their aponeuroses;
- inferiorly, the levator ani, coccygeus, transverse perineal, bulbospongiosus, ischiocavernosus, and anal sphincter muscles and their aponeuroses.

The pelvic organs are supported and held in place by the peritoneum, by ligaments containing contractile fibers (see below), and by muscles, aponeuroses, and other related connective tissues.

## MEANS OF CONNECTION

The system by which pelvic organs are connected or attached to one another is simpler than that of the abdomen. There are no omenta, mesenteries, nor double serous membranes. Connection is accomplished mainly by ligaments and various physiological mechanisms as described below.

### Ligaments

In the pelvis, ligaments contain contractile fibers. The degree of contractility is affected by general body tonus and by levels of certain hormones (particularly progesterone, and to a lesser extent estrogen). The position of the uterus varies according to stage of the menstrual cycle. We can treat the pelvic ligament system either by stretching (direct manipulation) or by increasing tonus (induction or active exercises).

Similar contractility is exhibited by the pelvic aponeuroses and space-filling tissues. The perineum seems to act like a sponge which can absorb or discharge fluids, tightening or slackening depending upon local or general factors which influence tonus. Actually, we believe that essentially all ligaments in the human body have contractile properties which can be modified by local or general factors; so far, however, we have been able to demonstrate this only for the pelvic ligaments.

### Reciprocal Tensions

As for all organs of the body, the pelvic organs are held against each other by reciprocal tension. The mast of a tent will remain vertical only if all the bracing-wires have equal tension. If a single wire is too loose or too tight, the equilibrium of the mast and all the other wires is disturbed. In the human body, a given restriction or injury can never be isolated; the consequences can be surprisingly far-reaching. A sprained ankle can have adverse effects on the bladder or uterus, as we shall see.

Good health can be viewed as effective compensation/adaptation by the body to its many stresses. Nonetheless, each stress leaves an indelible trace. When the individual's resistance is low, or there are too many accumulated traces, illness typically follows. For example, most cases of acute low back pain are triggered by seemingly trivial or innocuous movements. We believe that in these cases the area was *prepared* or *preprogrammed* for pain by cumulative previous stresses. Any trauma or abnormal tension can become part of the "memory" of a given organ or structure. Therefore, we must never overlook or neglect any articulation, however insignificant it may seem. In both evaluation and treatment, we must always think about the functioning of the whole body, not just an isolated part.

## Turgor Effect and Intracavitary Pressures

Turgor effect is the ability of an organ to occupy a maximal space within a given cavity, due to its elasticity and vascular pressure. Turgor effect in the pelvic organs results in tight space-filling. Because the organs are tightly packed, a surprisingly small amount of serous fluid is sufficient to allow proper sliding and cohesion of the organs and other structures.

The gas contained in the digestive organs contributes to turgor effect in the abdominal cavity. Gas contained in the small intestine influences the pelvic organs. It is easy to see how a spastic colon can push down on the bladder and stimulate the urethral sphincter. The urogenital organs do not produce gas; however, turgor effect is also affected by the presence of liquid. For example, the amount of urine in the bladder will influence the mobility of surrounding organs. A very full bladder will compress the other organs simply by an increase in volume.

The diaphragm has a strong influence on the abdominal organs. At greater distances, the effect of the diaphragm tends to diminish. However, we were surprised by the effects (revealed by fluoroscopy) of diaphragmatic movement on the bladder and uterus. With deep inhalation, the bladder may move downwards by 1.5cm. In patients with "paradoxical respiration," it may move downward during exhalation!

The peritoneum separates the pelvic cavity from the abdominal cavity, and plays an important role in distribution of intracavitary pressures. For this reason, it is very important to promptly diagnose and treat any peritoneal adhesion. The relationships between different intracavitary pressures can be summarized as follows:

- intravisceral pelvic pressure is greater than extracavitary pelvic pressure (the bladder is an exception; see below);
- extracavitary pelvic pressure is greater than peritoneal (abdominal) cavity pressure;
- peritoneal cavity pressure is greater than intrapulmonary pressure;
- intrapulmonary pressure is greater than pleural cavity pressure.

These relationships illustrate that the pelvic organs are essentially "suspended" from the abdominal parietal peritoneum. The peritoneum is, in turn, suspended from the diaphragm, which is suspended from the thorax. Thus, a pleuropulmonary restriction can easily affect pelvic organs via a chain of restrictions which we call a lesional chain (see *Visceral Manipulation II*, pp. 5-6). If a patient presents with a pleuropulmonary restriction in combination with pelvic congestion, and you treat only the latter, there is little chance of real improvement.

The effects of the diaphragm on pressures in the abdominal and pelvic cavities have been studied by Drye (1948). He measured intraperitoneal pressure in a supine female subject as 3cm $H_2O$. Pressures in a standing subject varied from 30cm $H_2O$ in the rectouterine pouch, to 8cm $H_2O$ in the epigastrium, to less than 5cm $H_2O$ in the subdiaphragmatic region. During such strenuous activities as coughing or sneezing, pressures in the pelvis can reach as high as 80cm $H_2O$.

As noted above, pressure inside the bladder behaves differently from that in other pelvic organs. In order for urine to collect, pressure in the bladder must remain low (approximately 10cm $H_2O$ at rest). If bladder pressure were higher than surrounding pelvic pressure, urine would not descend the ureters and would instead back up in the kidneys (hydronephrosis). During urination, of course, the situation changes. The openings to the ureters are shut off, the muscles of the bladder wall contract, pressure inside the bladder rises as high as 100cm $H_2O$, and urine passes out via the urethra.

## Transmission of Pressures

Pressure is transmitted by two systems: vertical/lateral transmission and inferior transmission *(Illustration 1-10)*.

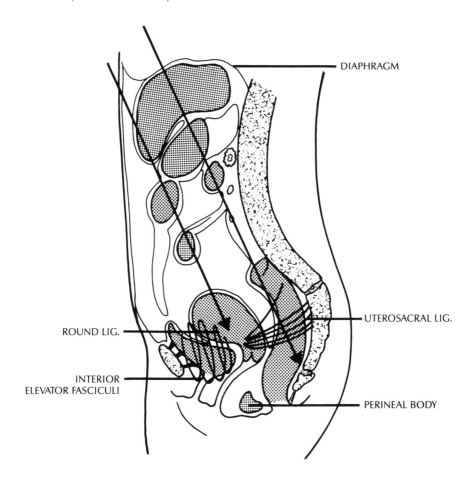

**Illustration 1-10**
Transmission of Pressures

VERTICAL / LATERAL TRANSMISSION: The organs of the abdomen and pelvis rest one upon the other to form a "visceral column." Because of gravity, pressure in this column is directed vertically downward and laterally against the bony/muscular walls. If the tonus of the muscular wall becomes deficient, the axis of vertical support changes and certain organs are subjected to less or more stress than usual. In the more-stressed organ, supporting muscles and ligaments are strained, circulatory and lymphatic vessels are compressed, and sensory nerve fibers are chronically stimulated. Fibrosis may develop as a defense against these abnormal pressures, and in turn prevent the organ from effectively retransmitting them.

INFERIOR TRANSMISSION: In the pelvic cavity, pressure is distributed via the perineal muscles and other subperitoneal tissues. Differential contraction of the muscles can lead to large variations in pressure which, in some cases, create structural restrictions. It is essential to have a supple perineum (not merely supple perineal muscles) which is able to expand and contract. Otherwise, the effort of coughing can contribute to cumulative damage of certain connective tissue or muscle fibers.

DIRECTION OF PRESSURES: As distance from the lungs in a downward direction increases, pressure increases. The pelvic organs support the weight of the abdominal organs and have less assistance from the "attraction" of the diaphragm. Pressures on the pelvic organs can be considerably increased by muscle contractions, coughing, sneezing, defecating, jogging, childbirth, and other strenuous activities.

The pelvic inlet is tilted forward to such an extent that abdominal pressure is directed mainly to the internal iliac fossae and iliopubic rami. Because of the dome-like shape of the visceral mass, the pressure coming from above distributes itself fairly evenly onto the perineum. In the healthy subject, the perineum is able to compensate for unusual pressure variations and to use its own tonus to partially counteract the pressure coming from above.

## Orifice-Closing Mechanisms

The perineal floor contains orifices for passage of the rectum, urethra, major vessels, etc. These openings represent "points of least resistance" to pressure. The striated muscles of the perineum must simultaneously enclose the pelvic cavity and allow opening of the orifices. Accordingly, the smooth muscle sphincters around a given orifice are usually contracted; when they relax, the orifice opens. In the case of the bladder, continence is assured as long as urethral pressure is greater than bladder pressure. If the striated or smooth muscles around a given orifice become weakened, the normal situation is disrupted and pressure from above (which tends to open the orifice) begins to dominate pressure from below (which tends to close it). This can lead not only to incontinence but also to a general weakening of the pelvic floor, which loses its ability to oppose the pressure from above. Without correction, the pelvic organs become more vertical and gradually migrate toward the orifices.

## Proper Confluence of Pelvic Pressures

For proper, even distribution of intrapelvic pressure, all the orifices (particularly their smooth muscle sphincters) must be correctly positioned (Illustration 1-11). The slightest downward displacement of the sphincters causes intrapelvic pressure to disrupt sphincter tonus instead of reinforcing or stimulating it.

As explained above, the pelvic floor is an elastic environment. Of the downward pressure from the visceral column, only the horizontal vector component helps keep the urethral and anal sphincters closed. When the pelvic floor is weakened, the vertical pressure component becomes predominant and opposes the closing of the sphincters.

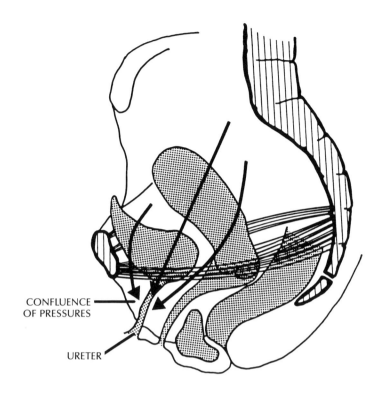

**Illustration 1-11**
Confluence of Pelvic Pressures

During normal perineal contraction, urethral pressure increases without modification of bladder or abdominal/pelvic pressures; this is the result of a lengthening of the urethra and active contraction of the external (voluntary) sphincter.

# Pathology of Movement

Our primary interest as osteopaths is in the mobility of structures. In this section, we will mention some of the lesions and restrictions which can affect mobility of the pelvic organs. We use the term **restriction** when an organ completely or partially loses its ability to move (either actively or passively). We use the term **adhesion** when an organ loses the ability to slide upon surrounding organs or structures.

## ETIOLOGY

Restrictions and adhesions arise from several different causes.

### Infection

Infections typically cause inflammation and exudation of the tissues involved. Resulting microadhesions or macroadhesions affect the elasticity of the tissues and production of serous fluid. The tissues or organ cannot slide normally, and retraction of scar tissue limits the amplitude of movement. Pathological anchor-points caused by scarring alter the organ's axis of movement, modifying its movements and those of neighboring structures.

Motility is the first type of movement to be affected, because of its small amplitude and weak force. When mobility is affected, the organ loses its normal tonicity and may become interdependent with an adjacent organ or even the pelvic wall. Rubbing of fibrosed tissues against neighboring tissues leads to irritation, which in turn stimulates the nervous system and causes vascular or visceral spasms. The immune defenses of an organ weaken as its mobility is lost, increasing its vulnerability to the numerous pathogenic agents present in the urogenital systems.

Frequent, minor infections produce scarring of which the patient may be totally unaware. To find and fix the associated microadhesions requires a highly skilled practitioner. Function of a sphincter may be reduced 30% or so because of nearby microadhesions. Even when microadhesion does not take place, viscosity of the organ's environment can be reduced. When such an organ is manipulated, it produces a characteristic crackling noise.

### Post-surgical Problems

A scar from surgery is like an iceberg in that only 10% of it is visible at the surface. Think about and investigate all the deeper levels which have been cut and sewn together! They do not have the same axis or direction as the superficial level. We shall see how to palpate a scar, using abdominal/vaginal mobility tests, in order to evaluate possible restrictions.

### Ligament Distention or Prolapse

These ligament injuries are the most visible, the easiest to detect, and the most difficult to treat. They result from loss of tonus of pelvic ligaments, which have contractile properties as discussed above. In *prolapse*, the ligaments no longer hold an organ in place, and it loses its normal connections to surrounding structures. This is comparable to luxation of a bony joint. In uterine prolapse, the cervix may be visible or even protrude from the vaginal orifice.

We have observed a greater tendency towards prolapse in longiline asthenic people. However, pregnancy and childbirth pose the greatest risk of urogenital prolapse. Removal of the baby by suction or forceps, without regard for the natural contractions, and a large episiotomy, favor collapse of the perineum and prolapse of the organs it supports. These factors, plus post-partum hypotonia and psychological depression, give the mother small chance of avoiding stress incontinence.

The probability of prolapse also increases with age, when tissues lose their elasticity and tonicity, and organs are progressively dragged downward by gravity.

### Visceral Spasms

The walls of hollow or tube-shaped organs contain longitudinal and circular smooth muscle fibers. These fibers may stay contracted for long periods of time if irritated. A common example of such "visceral irritability" is chronic contraction of the bladder wall.

In this situation, visceral fluid circulation is impaired, mobility is diminished, and motility almost disappears. Visceral spasms can be of direct or indirect origin:

- direct: local irritation from fibrous scar tissue, tumors, foreign bodies, infections, or adverse local effect of hormonal stimulus;
- indirect: reflex osteoarticular restrictions, lesional chains, peripheral or central neuropathy, systemic illness, or central hormonal imbalance.

## ENERGETIC PROBLEMS

### Desynchronization

One of the paradoxes of the body is that each organ has its own rhythm of motility, yet motility is a property of the whole body. No organ is autonomous; each has to function in a synchronized manner with its environment. When an organ is in spasm or otherwise impaired, its motility is altered and the rhythm and amplitude are diminished. In a sense, the organ becomes isolated. It no longer benefits from the motion of surrounding tissues; actually it opposes them. The organ requires more energy to continue functioning, which leads inevitably to exhaustion and illness.

### Vital Energy and Energy Cycles

The human body obtains energy from food. This energy is then consumed, converted, or stored in various ways. Each organ needs a certain amount of energy to function properly. A healthy organ consumes relatively little energy. In some cases, an organ uses too much energy—possibly even depriving other organs of the energy they need. Motility tests and local listening will reveal the culprit to us, even though symptoms of this energy imbalance may appear elsewhere. Many medical philosophies (most notably Oriental medicine) characterize illnesses in terms of exhaustion or transfer of energy. This approach is ignored by many Western practitioners, but we have found it helpful in many cases.

The liver, along with the hypothalamic-pituitary system, plays a key role in coordination of energy distribution and balance. It is well known that an athlete with a liver disorder is more liable to suffer from ligament or joint problems. Spring and autumn are the seasons when the liver is most vulnerable, and sprains are most frequent. We have no proof of a cause-effect relationship between these phenomena, but do not believe all our observations can be attributed to coincidence.

All people seem to contain a collection of internal physiological "clocks," with many different periodicities (daily, annual, monthly, etc.) We see examples of this frequently in our clinic. A patient may suffer from recurrent peptic ulcers for a year; the ulcers then disappear for five years (even though the patient's life-style and diet are unchanged), reappear for one year, disappear again, etc. After a few years of practice, most clinicians notice that they see the same illnesses in certain patients every equinox or solstice. The effect of many drugs varies depending on what hour of the day the drug is taken.

These physiological and other cycles of the human body and mind remain a great mystery. There have been explanations based on religion, astrology, genetics, hormones, cosmic forces, and much more. Our viewpoint, as always, is that *only the tissues know*. In our practice, we try to use a small but precise stimulation to solicit a reaction from the patient's body. If by this means we can facilitate or restore the body's own natural processes, our treatment is much more effective than if we tried to force the body to do something.

In females, tonus of the pelvic ligaments and muscles varies depending on stage of menstrual cycle, time of year, menopause, and many other factors. Stress incontinence is more frequent in the spring, and our treatments are least likely to have lasting benefit during this season.

# Treatment

Mobility and motility, discussed above in terms of evaluation techniques, can also be utilized for treatment of restrictions.

## MOBILITY

Use direct or indirect stretching to free fibrous, sclerosed, or adhered tissues and restore their original elasticity and tonicity. Your treatment should never "force" a tissue or create new irritations. If your treatment is too forceful or too prolonged the patient will probably experience a painful reaction. In this case, she should be instructed to return immediately and you should correctly treat the affected structure. The goal of osteopathy is to help the body heal itself. Treatment that is too strong or prolonged will not accomplish this purpose.

## MOTILITY

Use motility tests or listening for evaluation. Motility tests are performed with your hand on the patient's body, facing the organ to be tested. Apply pressure of 20-100 grams (slightly more than that used for checking craniosacral rhythm). Visualize the organ and its shape clearly and precisely. Don't try to feel any particular motion; be open to whatever you feel. Your hand should passively follow a slow motion (7 cycles per minute) of feeble amplitude, going back and forth around a neutral point. For most people it takes a long time of apprenticeship before they can become confident and skilled in feeling motility. Novices typically induce the motion, or end up testing a projection of their own motility or their own imagination.

For treatment, use induction to restore proper motility. Progressively accentuate the part of the cycle with greater amplitude and vitality until normal rhythm, frequency, and amplitude return. Often (not always) there is a *still point* and a release (see *Visceral Manipulation*, pp. 23-24).

We often use a technique between normal stretching and induction. Start out as if you were going to mobilize the tissues. From this point, perform local listening and then follow your fingers, gently and rhythmically, in the direction that you feel. Continue until you feel a release. The amount of force used is slightly more than in induction. This is a powerful technique useful in many situations, but does require considerable skill and finesse.

## TONICITY

Since the pelvic ligaments are contractile, their mechanoreceptors, tonoreceptors, and baroreceptors are very responsive to induction techniques. We mentioned an example

In which a retroverted uterus was corrected by approximately 30° simply by induction. Treating tonicity is an indirect way of affecting pelvic vascular and fluid systems. As we will explain later, pelvic tonicity can be reinforced by tonification of the perineum and its sphincters.

## METHODS OF TREATMENT

We generally treat our patients at monthly intervals and expect to see some improvement by the third session (of course, there are some exceptions). There is no point in administering a prolonged series of treatments if progress is obviously not being made. If you are not having success by the third session, refer the patient to some other type of therapy. If we do obtain success, after the third session we ask the patient to return after an interval of 3-4 months, then another 6 months. The body needs time to adapt and restore itself. Osteopathy does not replace the body's natural processes; it simply aids the body in a critical time or situation.

There is another reason for this regimen. We have observed repeatedly that when our treatments are successful the effects increase over time. That is, improvements in motion 3 or 4 weeks after treatment are greater than immediately after treatment. We believe that the nervous system plays a part in this phenomenon. When some area of the body is restricted for a long time, afferent nervous input to the relevant nuclei of the spinal cord and brain will diminish. In due course the central nervous system will "forget" the area in question, resulting either in some functional atrophy or that area being "left on." Our manipulations stimulate the local nervous system, leading to an increase in afferent transmission. Over time, this may recreate the normal afferent/efferent cycle and functioning.

We avoid the word "cure." We can certainly bring about relief, but there is no such thing as a complete cure. Illness is a complex phenomenon potentially affected by a multitude of factors (social, economic, genetic, psychological, etc.) over which we have no control. "Cure" is a static concept. The body and its health are constantly changing.

Likewise, we prefer the word "treat" to "heal." When you think in terms of "healing" another person you take on an unnatural, god-like role. It is as if the patient is defined only by her symptoms and nothing else. Also, since it is rare to permanently heal anyone, this type of attitude usually leads to a sense of failure. Do not exaggerate your own powers. The role of the osteopath is to develop knowledge of the human body and utilize that knowledge to solicit self-healing processes in the body. The more you learn about the background and environment of the patient, the better your chances of success.

There is some controversy about how long to wait after childbirth before attempting manipulation of the pelvic area. Most practitioners suggest waiting 4 to 6 weeks, to give the tissues reasonable opportunity to heal themselves. We prefer to wait until after the first menstrual period post-partum. The tissues of lactating mothers are quite difficult to work with. Of course, in cases of significant pain related to obstetrical procedures (e.g., episiotomy) it may be necessary to give treatment soon after childbirth, but effects will usually not be long-lasting.

# *Contraindications*

There are many situations in which urogenital manipulation is not advisable, or should be attempted only with caution.

## ABSOLUTE CONTRAINDICATIONS

PREGNANCY: For most women, this is one of the most important events in their lives. We have no proof that internal genital manipulation is harmful to the pregnant woman or the fetus, but we have no proof to the contrary either! Imagine the situation of a practitioner faced with a patient who miscarried after osteopathic manipulation, even if this were not the direct cause. We have treated over 3,000 patients without ever encountering this situation; on the other hand, we know of a patient who was treated by another practitioner and miscarried 48 hours later. She is still convinced there was a cause-and-effect relationship between the two events. We also oppose the use of any internal technique designed to induce abortion, even at early stages of pregnancy.

VIRGINITY: For obvious reasons, you should not attempt internal genital manipulation on a female virgin.

UNACCOMPANIED MINORS: Never treat a minor unless she is accompanied by one or both parents. We often ask young patients to come accompanied by a husband or friend.

METRORRHAGIA: Loss of blood other than at the time of normal menstrual flow is abnormal. We recommend that any woman with this symptom undergo a complete gynecological exam by her primary medical practitioner or a gynecologist before any osteopathic manipulation takes place. The most frequent cause of such bleeding in a young woman is pregnancy. Other possible causes, in both young and older women, are fibromas, neoplasms of the cervix or body of the uterus, infection, endometriosis, uterine polyps, ovarian tumors, and hormonal dysfunctions. Even a trace of blood, if unexplained, warrants a complete gynecological exam.

ANY ABNORMAL, SUDDEN, OR ACUTE PAIN: Such pain, either described by the patient or provoked by palpation, is cause for concern. Suggest a gynecological exam in the near future. Sudden and acute pains are discussed in the "Differential Diagnosis" section of chapter 4 below.

ANY INDURATION OR MASS: Be alert for lateral or posterior indurations or masses, sometimes filling the pouches. When these are sensitive, even if not painful, they may represent such problems as salpingitis, adnexitis, ectopic pregnancy, tumors, or ovarian cysts. Similarly, always monitor the patient carefully for any change in her general condition. Be alert for such "red flags" as fever, weight loss, adenopathy, localized foul odor, or dermatological lesions. If these are unexplained or not previously documented, try to obtain a diagnosis.

AFTER RADIATION THERAPY: Normal clotting mechanisms are impaired in these cases and internal urogenital manipulation may provoke local hemorrhage. We witnessed one such case in which the bleeding was very difficult to stop.

# RELATIVE CONTRAINDICATIONS

These cautions are less emphatic. The following signs suggest that we differentiate or modify urogenital manipulations, but do not prohibit them outright.

EXPLAINED TRACES OF BLOOD: Documented endometriosis is the best example. Since
there is chronic bleeding of the uterine mucosa, direct or forceful techniques may increase
bleeding and are therefore not advisable. On the other hand, *functional* manipulations,
in the direction of listening, are recommended since they tend to decrease local spasms
and improve local venous and lymphatic circulation.

LOCAL INFECTIONS: In some cases where conventional medical treatment has been
attempted and failed, local manipulations may enhance resistance to the infectious agent.
Osteopathic treatment alone can never cure an infection; be sure that standard medical
treatments (e.g., antibiotics) are applied first, and work with them. It is important to treat
any pelvic infection promptly, since it may have long-lasting effects on the ovaries or
uterine tubes. Principal signs of local pelvic infection are:

- inguinal adenopathy,
- local hypersensitivity or pain,
- pruritus,
- dermatological marks,
- foul vaginal odors,
- presence of blood on the glove following pelvic exam.

The latter can also be simply the result of irritating sensitive mucosa or something more serious (e.g., cervical cancer). In general, our manipulations should not cause
bleeding.

PRESENCE OF AN INTRAUTERINE DEVICE: Inexperienced practitioners might potentially alter the position of an I.U.D. when approaching the uterine cervix via either the
vagina or rectum. We have never encountered this situation ourselves. However, imagine
how you would deal with a patient with an I.U.D. who became pregnant a few weeks
after internal manipulation.

HYPERSENSITIVITY OR SLIGHT PAIN ON PALPATION: Under "Absolute Contraindications," we mentioned abnormal and acute pain provoked by palpation. Less intense
types of pain should make us cautious and conservative in our treatment. If there is hypersensitivity or slight pain which *increases* in intensity during treatment, you should aban-
don internal manipulation or reconsider your tactics. The cause is often sloppy or
inappropriate manipulation, endometriosis, or atrophied genital tissue. Because of the
quality of the genital tissues, internal manipulation properly performed should, in general,
rapidly decrease local pain. Certainly any increase is not normal.

Pain provoked by vaginal exam can have different causes depending on the depth
where pain is first perceived; these usually correspond to localization of dyspareunia (pain
on intercourse). Pain on initial penetration can be due to vaginismus, perineal lacera-
tion, or urethritis. Pain midway can reflect partial rupture of the levators, bladder inflammation (trigonitis), or vaginal dystrophy. Pain at the end of penetration can reflect tearing
or rupture of the uterosacral ligaments (this pain rarely stays localized, but rapidly radiates into the abdominal or renal areas), endometriosis (particularly during and just after
menstruation), or problems of the uterine cervix (benign or otherwise).

# *The Lesional Chain*

For the osteopath, investigation and treatment of the immediate symptoms are not sufficient. Although the patient may present with stress incontinence, dyspareunia, uterine restriction, or whatever, you need to obtain a complete case history and carry out a thorough evaluation. The more complete your information, the better your chance of effective treatment.

In principle, the osteopath should ignore secondary symptoms and search for the real, underlying pathology. Realistically, though, it is often sufficient to just be a little "less secondary." Analysis of a lesional chain means delving into the patient's pathological history. But many questions always remain unanswered. So many pathological events were seemingly harmless at the time and either unnoticed or promptly forgotten. Other events may be recorded only in the "memory" of the genes.

The search for ultimate cause is like the philosopher's stone—a goal which, at some level, we know to be unachievable. This knowledge, far from discouraging us, simply obliges us to look further. Osteopathy, the science of motion, can only work if its practitioners are also mobile and flexible.

When dealing with urogenital problems, one must examine all parts of the body which could conceivably have some causative association with the restriction. The most "likely suspects" (based on our clinical experience) are listed below.

- Skull: The urogenital system is under the direct influence of the hypothalamic-pituitary axis. Urogenital problems are frequently associated with restrictions of the sphenobasilar joint, or occipitoparietal and occipitomastoid sutures.
- Cervical spine, clavicle, T1, and first rib: Restrictions here are also common in patients with urogenital problems. These segments have effects on the stellate ganglion and thyroid gland, and thereby on hormones affecting the urogenital system.
- Thoracic spine: Aside from T1, the urogenital area is most closely associated with T7 and T11 due to its innervation. With disorders of the kidneys (e.g., nephritis), T7 is usually restricted.
- Lumbar spine, sacrum, and coccyx: These segments (especially the coccyx) are typically affected in urogenital disorders.
- Lower limbs: Almost every urogenital restriction is reflected in the leg or foot. The most frequent restrictions are those of the inferior tibiofibular joint, navicular, and fifth metatarsal. To reinforce this fact, we often ask students to begin treatment of urogenital problems by manipulating the foot.

Using fluoroscopy, we have documented a motion of the bladder associated with pressure on the inferior aspect of the navicular; similar pressure on the inferior cuboid had no effect. Sprains of the foot or ankle often lead to urogenital problems; conversely, a urogenital problem can render a leg or foot joint more susceptible to injury. Interestingly, we very rarely find such associations of the forearm or hand with other parts of the body. Perhaps these are actually rare; or perhaps the upper limbs are a relative "blind spot" for us.

## CASE HISTORY

In this section, we shall describe an actual case history which illustrates the route taken by a typical lesional chain. We are by no means implying that all our cases have such satisfactory results!

Mrs. X, 48 years old, complained of a chronic right supracondylar knee pain. She had three children; the first childbirth was laborious and difficult. She was in good general health aside from some dyspareunia and episodic stress incontinence. History and radiological examination were unremarkable. She was surprised that we asked her about urogenital problems when she came to see us about knee pain. Osteopathic tests revealed:

- abnormal tension of the posterior fasciculi of the right iliolumbar ligaments;
- a painful restriction of the sacrococcygeal joint on anterior flexion. Mrs. X. had never experienced coccygeal pain in her life, had no memory of any related fall, and was surprised by the pain caused by the test. We had to perform the test several times to convince her that it was not the (slight) pressure of our fingers which caused the pain.
- a very fixed navicular (she did remember an ankle strain incurred and untreated 15 years previously);
- anterior flexion of the bladder and uterus;
- Sensitivity of the right knee in the medial femoral region, with redness and slight swelling of the cutaneous projection of the medial collateral ligament;
- a severely restricted knee joint.

### Treatment

During the first session, we treated the sacrococcygeal joint. When this was released, the restrictions of the right iliolumbar ligaments and navicular disappeared. During the second session one month later, using direct manipulation and induction, we freed all the anterior attachment systems of the bladder (median and medial umbilical ligaments, and pubovesical ligaments). Two weeks after this, the knee pain had slightly diminished. During the third session (one month after the second), we stretched the inguinal canal and the trochanteric muscles, which were slightly spasmed in compensation for the release of more primary restrictions. The knee pain subsequently dissipated entirely, along with (more gradually) the dyspareunia and incontinence.

We have followed Mrs. X for over 10 years and she has remained in generally good health. There are some radiographic signs of arthritis in the right knee, but no pain or disability. We believe these signs may result from a thoracic problem.

### Analysis

At this point, you may be asking yourself: How can a right supracondylar knee pain be treated via the coccyx and bladder, without ever touching the knee itself? We also wondered about this and conducted much fruitless literature searching until one day when, rereading our "bible," the topographical anatomy text of Testut and Jacob (1927), we noticed that:

- the genitofemoral nerve, after its passage through the inguinal canal, sends a branch to the medial part of the knee capsule, exactly where our patient was experiencing pain;

- the round ligaments also pass through the inguinal canal. Therefore, when the bladder and uterus were fixed anteriorly, fibrosis of these ligaments mechanically irritated the genitofemoral nerve.

We concluded that this mechanical excitation produced a neuritis which in turn led to capsulitis of the knee joint. Other hypotheses are no doubt possible, but we must admit that this chain of restrictions is satisfying to us!

## CONCLUSION

Human organisms are under considerable restraints and pressures. When a structure loses its elasticity and distensibility, it can become dissociated from the incessant motion of the surrounding tissues. These motions are due to the diaphragm, skeletal movement, heart, primary respiratory motion, and local peristalsis. We do not believe that any fibrosis can be without consequences. The slightest disturbance of a tissue destabilizes the reciprocal tension of all the supple elements of the organism in the same manner that a piece missing in an enormous house of cards destroys its balance.

The multifactorial bombardment of a structure, repeated millions of times, is at the beginning asymptomatic. But soon small symptoms appear and illness develops. Usually there is a comment like, "She was so well yesterday!"

As osteopaths, we often see only the end result of a complex lesional chain which began far in the past. In some cases, like that of Mrs. X, we are still able to obtain good results. In other cases, we are not so lucky. Ideally, we would like to be able to intervene at the beginning of a potential lesional chain. Osteopathy should not be a treatment of "last resort." Our practice should not depend upon the failure of other therapies. Osteopathy can, and should, be a form of preventive medicine.

# Chapter Two:
## The Bladder

# Table of Contents

# *The Bladder*

T here are unique difficulties in dealing with stress incontinence. Whereas certain illnesses may give the patient vague feelings of heroism or stoicism, incontinence gives the patient a feeling of regression, of shame, of being "dirty" like a child. The incontinent woman may feel alone with this problem, and attempt to hide it from those around her. Some of our patients have successfully concealed their problem from their own husbands for ten years or more. These women use products such as absorbent powders, deodorants, special pants, and douches, often pointlessly. Accurate statistics are hard to come by, but we would estimate that at least 40% of women suffer from some degree of incontinence. Sometimes this problem results from simple hormonal disorders, and can be easily treated or even disappear by itself. Some cases are much more difficult to treat.

As with all practitioners, we began with good results in a few patients for which we did not know the exact explanation. Moved by the complaints of these patients we wanted to have a better understanding so that we could be even more effective. This is part of the reason why this book was written.

We remember the case of a professional tennis player who, with each racket stroke, lost urine. Her solution was to drink as little as possible, and avoid getting close to other people. Naturally, this led to increasing isolation, to the point where she stopped training and going to tournaments. When she first consulted us she was severely dehydrated, depressed, afflicted by buildup of toxic compounds in the body, and scheduled to undergo a Marshall-Marchetti-Krantz type of cystopexy. Fortunately, osteopathic treatment successfully reduced the incontinence, and she was able to return to the professional circuit without surgery.

Again, we wish that osteopaths were more often viewed as doctors of first resort rather than last resort. We are strong believers in avoiding needless surgery. Manipulation should be among the treatments considered first for stress incontinence.

This chapter is concerned mainly with incontinence, and to a lesser degree with cystitis and repeated cystalgia. These are all common and psychologically oppressive disorders. They are primarily afflictions of women, especially those who have undergone pregnancy and childbirth; we have seen hundreds of cases of this type. The few men who have consulted us tend to come for neurological re-education rather than osteopathic treatment.

We will focus on the bladder and associated structures in this chapter. However, we remind the reader again to always look at the whole body, not an isolated part, when treating a patient.

# *Anatomy*

We will briefly describe the anatomy of the bladder and its environment here. Thorough understanding of basic anatomy is essential for understanding of physiology and pathology. This is not an exhaustive description; please keep your standard anatomy texts ready for reference.

## VESICAL CAVITY

The cavity within which the bladder lies is determined by the pelvic walls, various muscles and ligaments, and other organs *(Illustration 2-1)*. Specifically, the cavity consists of the following elements:

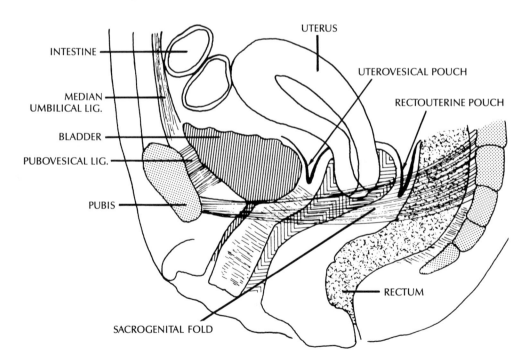

**Illustration 2-1**
Vesical Cavity

- superiorly: superior vesical pouch, small intestine, and sometimes the fundus of the uterus (depending upon its position);
- anteriorly: pubis, its ligaments and muscular attachments, and peritoneum;
- posteriorly: cervix/isthmus portion of uterus, and vagina;
- inferiorly: urethra, vagina, space-filling subperitoneal tissue, internal obturator muscle, piriformis muscle, and other parts of the perineum;
- laterally: the lateral edges of the peritoneum curl back to form a hammock-shaped structure called the tendinous arch of the pelvic fascia (also known as the lateral true ligament of the bladder), which blends into the anterior layer of the broad ligaments.

## ADJACENT STRUCTURES AND THEIR RELATIVE LOCATION

Positions and relationships of the structures described below vary from person to person. The following are intended as "average" guidelines (Illustration 2-2). Do not be surprised when you encounter exceptions.

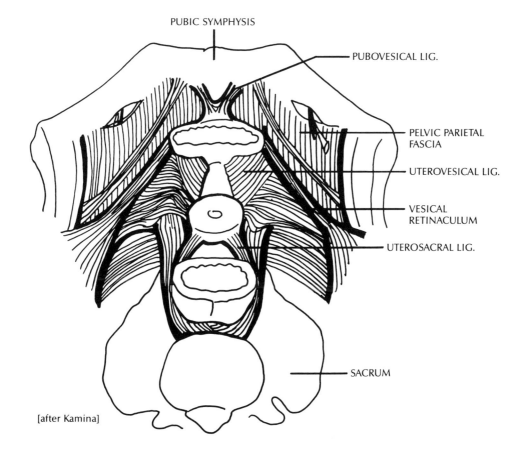

**Illustration 2-2**
Bladder: Means of Connection

The **peritoneum** adheres strongly to the vertex of the bladder. Although some workers deny that it has a significant suspensory role, our experience shows that a peritoneal adhesion can have definite adverse effects on bladder mobility and diaphragmatic attraction.

The **median and medial umbilical ligaments** function as a fascia joining the bladder to the umbilicus and continuing to the liver via the falciform ligament. They suspend the apex of the bladder and are important for mobilization. So far, however, we have not been able to document by fluoroscopy that stretching these ligaments has any significant effect on the bladder. The median umbilical ligament (the remnant of the urachus) is found on a line going from the umbilicus to the vesical apex, just underneath the skin and on the anterior parietal peritoneum, and is covered by the umbilicoprevesical aponeurosis. The medial umbilical ligaments are on two oblique lines running from the umbilicus to the vesical horns, on each side of the median umbilical ligament.

The **vesical fascia and tendinous arch of the pelvic fascia** are primarily anterior. They go from the umbilicus to the pubovesical ligaments, to the parietal pelvic fascia and, lastly, to the uterovesical ligaments or internal pillars of the bladder. They continue as the pubovesicals.

The **pubovesical and pubo-urethral ligaments** are comprised partly of the muscular fasciculi of the external layer of the detrusor (muscle of the bladder wall). They run from the posterior side of the pubic symphysis to the bladder, neck of the bladder, and urethra, and are connected to the vesicovaginal fascia. They need to be strong but also allow for bladder neck mobility inferiorly and posteriorly. The pubovesical ligaments are found at the point of contact between the posterior high and middle parts of the pubic symphysis and the anterior neck and body part. The pubo-urethral ligaments are located at the point of contact between the posteroinferior part of the pubic symphysis and the anterior labia.

The **posterior attachment system** is a fold coming from the parametrium (the dense inferior part of the broad ligaments) and sides of the vagina. The superior or uterovesical fasciculi of this system also contain fibers of the detrusor and form the vesical pillars. The interior fasciculi correspond to the vesicovaginal fascia.

The **vesical base** provides firm support and attachment for the bladder. The cervicotrigonal region is anchored to the pelvic floor by numerous fibers. It is supported by space-filling subperitoneal tissue and the sacrogenital folds which connect the bladder to the uterus, rectum, and sacrum. It rests upon the anterior wall of the vagina, to which it is linked by connective tissue folds which form the vesicovaginal septum. The perineum upon which the vesical base rests consists of the levator ani, internal obturator, ischiocavernosus, and bulbocavernosus muscles and associated aponeuroses. Injury to any of these muscles or fasciae can restrict mobility of the bladder. Note that the most important of these structures surround the obturator window.

The **vesical apex** is behind the pubic symphysis. The more urine the bladder contains, the more the apex projects above the crest of the symphysis.

The **neck of the bladder and trigone** are located approximately 2.5cm behind the pubis, about two-thirds of the way down that bone.

The **uterine cervix** corresponds to the posteroinferior side of the bladder and the trigone.

The **vagina** is 7-8cm in length. On its pelvic lateral portion (upper two-thirds), the finger touches the parametrium and urethra 1.5cm outside the lateral vaginal pouch. For the peritoneal portion, from top to bottom, the finger touches the internal fasciculi of the levator ani, pelvic and middle perineal aponeuroses, deep transverse muscle, constrictor of the vulva, and vestibulovaginal bulb. The vaginal septum is 6-8mm thick.

The **round ligaments** are 10-12cm long and 3-6mm in diameter. They are both distensible and contractile.

The **perineal body** is the hard fibrous mass felt when the region between the vulva and vagina is pressed superiorly.

In summary, the reader should note that the bladder's attachment system has numerous fibers in common with the detrusor (via the pubovesical and pubo-urethral ligaments), uterovesical fascia, and vesical pillars. This explains in part the reactions of the bladder to stretching of these ligaments. One can also visualize a muscular/apon-eurotic "chain" which links the bladder to the liver above and to the sacrum below via the falciform ligament, median umbilical ligament, prevesical fascia, fibers of the detru-sor, internal pillars of the bladder, and sagittal peritoneal folds. Because of this chain, manipulations of the liver can affect the bladder, and vice versa. The pubovesical and pubo-urethral ligaments insert themselves into the levator ani and obturator muscles, suggesting another possible lesional chain.

## SLIDING SURFACES

Our manipulations of the bladder depend on knowledge of its sliding surfaces. Our defibrosing action should be concentrated on areas where the bladder slides upon other organs and tissues. Despite its extraperitoneal position, the bladder has numerous con-tiguous relationships with the peritoneum. Specifically, it articulates:

- superiorly with the peritoneum, which is always assigned a negligible suspen-sory role by anatomists and surgeons except during a cystopexy. However, a peritoneal restriction can disturb the whole vesical axis and thus oppose satis-factory physiological movement. The bladder articulates with the intestinal loops and the pelvic colon via the peritoneum.
- anteriorly with the uterus (depending upon its position) and broad ligaments, and lower down with the anterior parietal peritoneum, prevesical space, and pubovesical ligaments;
- posteriorly, the very bottom of the bladder and trigonal region articulate with the uterine cervix/isthmus region via the vesicovaginal septum and, lower down, with the vagina via the vesicovaginal fascia;
- posterolaterally with the vesical fascia, lower part of the broad ligaments, parametrium, perineal muscles, and urethra.

# *Normal Bladder Physiology*

The distal part of the urinary system is designed to ensure that the bladder can gradually fill up, hold a certain volume of urine, and periodically allow urination. Depend-ing upon the situation, pressure within the urethra will be higher or lower than that in the bladder. During voluntary urination, the internal and external urethral sphincters relax, the detrusor contracts, and urethral pressure becomes lower than bladder pressure. This system is regulated by complex somatic and autonomic innervation.

Intravesical pressure always remains low (10-25cm $H_2O$ depending on bladder tonus) despite the presence of urine. This facilitates entrance of urine from the ureters, and maintenance of a relatively higher pressure in the urethra. When urinary volume approaches 350ml, stretching of collagen fibers in the bladder wall stimulates associated proprioceptors, leading to de-inhibition of the detrusor via a spinal reflex mechanism. When somatic (voluntary) control is combined with this autonomic reflex, the detrusor contracts strongly, intravesical pressure rises briefly to 50-100cm $H_2O$, the sphincters relax, and urine leaves the body via the urethra.

## OCCLUSION OF THE BLADDER NECK

The neck of the bladder has a "doubled-laced" occlusive system resulting from the orientation of the external fibers of the detrusor *(Illustration 2-3)*. The posterior lace corresponds to Hutch's "base plate," and the anterolateral and inferior laces to the loop of the detrusor which surrounds the internal urethra opening (Hutch, 1967). The fibers of the pubovesical muscle surround the posterior part of this opening and contribute to closing of the internal sphincter. These muscle fibers are supplied by a rich venous system in the urethral submucosa which appears to be a factor in continence.

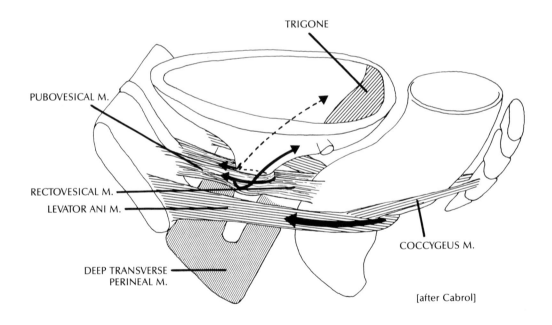

**Illustration 2-3**
Occlusion of Bladder Neck

This periurethral system is capable of great distention. The erectile tissue is like an elastic cushion for the surrounding perineal muscles. This may explain the rapid appearance of incontinence often observed a few months after menopause. Filling of the bladder triggers a beta reflex leading to relaxation of the detrusor, and an alpha reflex leading to contraction of the fibers around the urethral opening. The "base plate," under tension, moves the vertex of the trigone (and thus the posterior side of the neck) forward. The lace of the detrusor, during contraction, pulls the anterior side of the neck backward.

The occlusive effect is added to the high pressure within the urethra, which is related to urethral diameter, parietal pressure, and length of the urethra. We use urethral stretching to increase reciprocal pressure and tonoreceptor phenomena.

The role of the external (voluntary) urethral sphincter is somewhat controversial. Present evidence suggests that it has a negligible effect on continence during rest. It may be more important during physical effort, coughing, and sneezing.

## URETHRAL PRESSURE

Pressure in the urethra is low at the internal meatus (i.e., where the urethra exits the bladder), highest in the middle third, and declines again approaching the external meatus. Urethral pressure is controlled mainly by smooth muscles. It can also be influenced by the vascular plexus of the submucosa. E.g., Raz (1972) reported that urethral pressure diminished approximately 30% after clamping of the internal iliac arteries.

Some important and reproducible factors affecting urethral pressure are as follows:

- when the bladder is empty, urethral pressure is minimal;
- standing causes a significant increase in pressure;
- lengthening of the urethra increases urethral pressure (up to 40%). We utilize this in manipulation when we stretch fibrosed periurethral structures.
- contraction of the perineum increases urethral pressure but without modifying bladder or pelvic pressures. The increase is due to active contraction of the external urethral sphincter and stretching of the urethra. Susset (1976) reported that the length of the urethra was increased 0.5-1.0cm in this way.

Our experience shows that if the perineum is not sufficiently elastic or contractile, modification of urethral pressure through changing the length of the urethra is more difficult, and incontinence may result.

When abdominal/pelvic pressure increases, occlusion of the bladder neck must be reinforced in order to avoid incontinence. An increase in pelvic pressure is transferred to the proximal part of the urethra found above the pelvic floor. In response, the external sphincter contracts first, followed by the internal sphincter. With intense muscular effort, the perineum and all the pelvic muscles contract at the same time as the two sphincters.

During coughing and sneezing, elevated abdominal/pelvic pressure is accompanied by increased pressure in the bladder and proximal urethra. Above all, passive transfer of abdominal pressure at the level of the proximal urethra is what reinforces urethral pressure. Green (1975) believes that optimal transfer of pressure is assured by the periurethral tissues, and the vesico-urethral angle is important. We have found it helpful to pay attention to release of periurethral fibroses. Putting the pubo-urethral ligaments under pressure tends to oppose the effects of strenuous effort. In this context, we can refer to a suspensory system of the urethra.

In conclusion, with a slackening of the vesical base or pelvic floor, an increase of abdominal pressure is transferred more to the bladder than to the urethra. That is, pressure within the bladder increases without a corresponding increase within the urethra, and the occlusive system of the bladder neck loses its efficiency. The occlusive effects of the pubovesical, rectovesical, levator ani (both pubic and iliac portions), and deep transverse perineal muscles are all diminished.

## URINATION

As long as urethral pressure is higher than bladder pressure, urine will stay in the bladder. In urination provoked by bladder distention, the drop in urethral pressure precedes contraction of the detrusor and collapse of the bladder floor by several seconds. This pressure drop occurs in the proximal and middle urethra, not the distal portion which is more affected by movement of the perineum. The fibers of the internal (autonomic) urethral sphincter are derived from the detrusor. When they contract, a groove appears in the base of the bladder. The base extends posteriorly into the pubovesical muscle, which reinforces this effect. The fibers of the external (voluntary) sphincter are derived from perineal muscles.

### Role of the Nervous System

The role of the nervous system in urination is very complex. A detailed discussion of this would go far beyond the proper role of this book. Still, as osteopaths we need to always consider how the nervous system interplays with the structures and functions we deal with. Here only the most important circuits are listed. We encourage you to study more so you will be able to appreciate this wonderful mechanism:

- fronto-pons-mesencephalic circuit: this can be tested by asking the patient if she is capable of voluntarily inhibiting the contractions of the detrusor.
- brain stem circuit: this goes from the brain stem to the sacral centers and then on to the bladder and urethra.
- detrusor circuit: this involves the pudendal motor nucleus and its effect on the striated sphincter.
- cortex circuit: this contains a link from the cortex to the pudendal motor nucleus and then to the striated sphincter.

At present, as always, there remain many uncertainties dealing with the different reflexes that involve urination. These issues will continue to divide physiologists for some time. We need to be cognizant of the various possibilities for they can be helpful in particular patients.

## CONCLUSION

The system for occlusion of the bladder neck depends on structures of the bladder base, and the tonicity and position of the bladder. Urethral pressure depends on proper functioning of smooth muscles, striated muscles, reciprocal pressures, and the parietal vascular system. Tiny restrictions of the bladder area that affect the motion of the neck by only 1-2mm can lead to stress incontinence. At rest, urethral pressure is far from its maximal value; this "reserve capacity" enables it to cope with considerable increases in bladder pressure. Bladder and urethral pressures and position are regulated by a variety of physical and neuronal factors which are not yet completely understood. In general, autonomic control of urination can be overridden by voluntary control.

We have found that fibrosis, hypotonia, or loss of elasticity in the tissues of the bladder/perineal region tend to have the following adverse effects:

- ability of the urethra to change length is reduced;
- the perineum loses its ability to balance pressures and reinforce the urethra;
- the spongy vascular periurethral tissue becomes non-functional;
- the sphincters lose their occlusive ability.

## Stress Incontinence

The bladder has an anchorage system with two components: anterior and posterolateral *(Illustration 2-4)*. The anterior anchorage is supported by the perineal body and consists of the interior fasciculi of the levator ani and the muscular/connective tissue attached to the inferior half of the vagina. This anchorage is active and elastic. The posterolateral anchorage consists of the parametrium and uterosacral ligaments, and is more passive and solid.

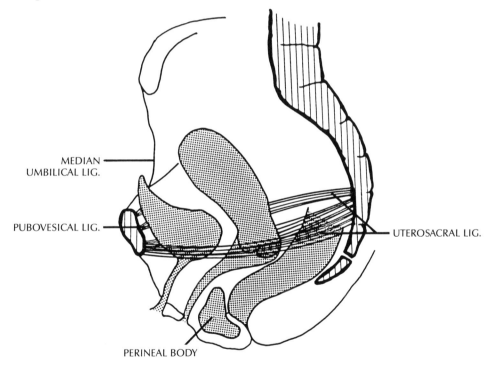

MEDIAN UMBILICAL LIG.

PUBOVESICAL LIG.

UTEROSACRAL LIG.

PERINEAL BODY

**Illustration 2-4**
Bladder Anchorage System

## INTRAPELVIC VISCERAL MOVEMENTS

Huguier et al. (1968) studied vesical movements using colpocystography. They evaluated pushing movements (for deliberate urination), and retention movements (for

conscious retention of urine). We extended these studies for evaluation of bladder movement during vigorous diaphragm contraction, coughing, lying position, standing position,
perineal contraction, contractions of the abductors, adductors, rotators, etc. This approach
enabled us to document and improve the effects of our osteopathic manipulations of the
bladder.

During retention movements, the anterior bladder anchorage contracts while the
posterolateral anchorage does not change. This increases the urethrovesical angle (urethral cap) and uterovaginal angle (vaginal cap). The rectum also forms a rectal cap. All
these angles have an anterior vertex.

During pushing movements, the anterior anchorage is released and the urethral
and vaginal caps disappear. The vesical base and uterine cervix/isthmus region move
slightly posteroinferiorly and press against the upper half of the vagina. The latter presses
upon the rectum and in this way shuts the rectouterine pouch. The levators pull the
lower half of the vagina forward *(Illustration 2-5)*. The rectal cap does not change because
the rectal ampule restricts it.

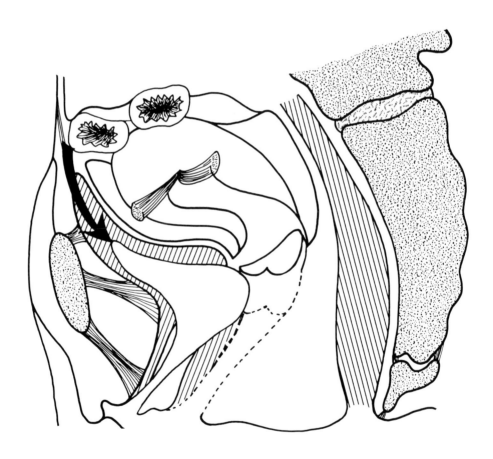

**Illustration 2-5**
Pushing Movement of Bladder

This movement takes place if the force is directed to an anteflexed and anteverted uterus. It is actually the uterus which transfers the force to the posterior bladder; the bladder then transfers it to the anterior vagina. With a retroverted uterus, or a restriction of the pelvic suspensory or support mechanisms, normal balance and pressure transmission are disrupted.

## CLASSIFICATION AND PATHOLOGY

The posterior urethrovesical angle is normally about 30° from the vertical. In some types of incontinence, it becomes greater than 45° with pushing effort. Loss of the posterior urethrovaginal angle results from weakness of the bladder neck and inadequate support by the levator muscles.

Normally, the bladder neck remains shut, its edges pressed together by action of the internal sphincter. The bladder neck does not normally descend below a horizontal

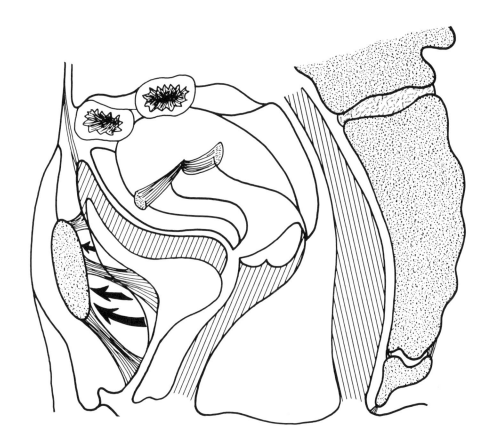

**Illustration 2-6**
Type A Incontinence

plane drawn from the inferior end of the pubic symphysis. A chronic opening in the bladder neck indicates failure of the internal sphincter.

Stress incontinence has traditionally been classified into three types: type A (anterior), type P (posterior), and mixed type. Type P is the most common.

## Type A Incontinence

In this type *(Illustration 2-6)*, the anterior bladder and urethral walls are fixed by adhesion or sclerosis to such an extent that, even with effort, the bladder remains pressed against the pubis. The loss of elasticity of the suspensory tissues at the junction of the urethra and bladder causes a form of dissociation, i.e., the bladder neck is dissociated from its two edges. The integrity of the junction is compromised, either because of poor support of the posterior bladder neck, or because the anterior aspect is fixed.

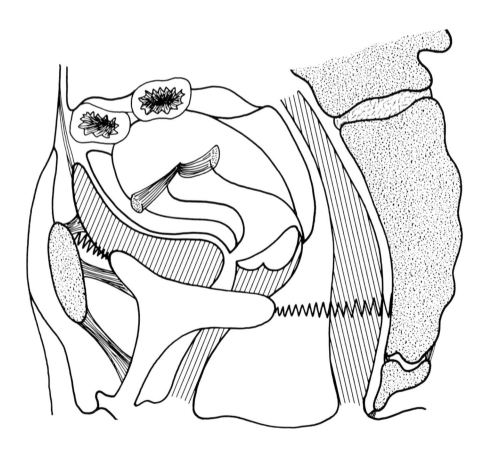

**Illustration 2-7**
Type P Incontinence

## Type P Incontinence

In type P stress incontinence *(Illustration 2-7)*, the posterolateral attachment system (sacrogenital fold, parametrium) slackens and the bladder collapses. The bladder neck/urethra junction moves outside the pressure enclosure of the abdomen and pelvis (see below). Because of this movement, transfer of abdominal pressure to the proximal urethra takes place inappropriately or not at all.

On colpocystography, the bladder is very mobile; with effort, its base moves posteroinferiorly. When the bladder neck is outside the abdominal pressure enclosure, pressure in the bladder predominates over sphincter pressure, interfering with normal continence.

Weakening of the posterior anchorage system lowers the vaginal dome, which brings the bladder along with it. The bladder floor is laterally contiguous with the vagina via the vesical pillars which lengthen the tendinous arch of the pelvic fascia. The vaginal dome and uterine neck essentially comprise a single organ which is held up by this arch, the parametrium, and the uterosacral ligaments. When these elements are distended or torn, they invite prolapse of the bladder.

## Mixed Type Incontinence

This combination of types A and P is the most severe but also, fortunately, the rarest type. We should note that these classifications are based solely on position. In osteopathy (as opposed to surgery) we are more concerned with motion than position, so this type of diagnosis may not be particularly helpful to us.

## Pathology

Information on bladder position is generally based on colpocystography. We must be cautious in interpreting these tests, since some entirely continent patients have abnormal colpocystograms. When suspension and support of the bladder are compromised, the fibers of the internal sphincter become incorrectly oriented and less functional. Faulty transfer of abdominal/pelvic pressure, however, is the factor having the greatest adverse effect.

Paradoxically, in some women with stress incontinence urination is not always facilitated. Certain prolapses cause a bend in the urethra which interferes with normal discharge of urine. Some women suffering from a prolapse become incontinent only after cystopexy. Prolapsed viscera become positioned under the urethra/bladder junction or the urethra, resulting in transmission to the proximal urethra of elevated pressure from pushing effort. With a urethrocystocele, pressure during urination is weaker, urethral resistance is increased, and the urination process is prolonged and accompanied by abdominal pushing.

## Abdominal Pressure Enclosure

According to Enhörning (1961), urinary incontinence with effort occurs only when the proximal urethra is outside the abdominal enclosure *(Illustration 2-8)*. In this situation, the urethra is not appropriately affected by increased abdominal pressure. We think that an additional factor here is that fibrosed or sclerosed periurethral and perivesical tissues (e.g., sequelae of an infection from childbirth or surgery) lose their mechanical distensibility and can no longer properly ameliorate or distribute the pressure.

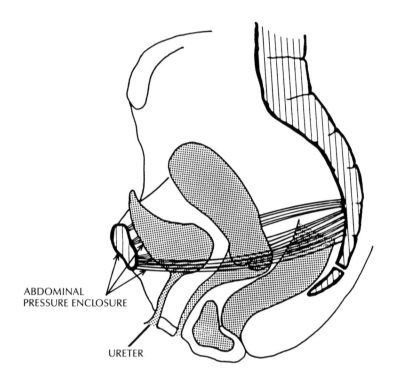

**Illustration 2-8**
Abdominal Pressure Enclosure

Other authors emphasize the chronic opening of the bladder neck and weakening of the internal sphincter. This prevents normal transmission of pressures and shifts responsibility for continence entirely to the external sphincter and pelvic floor. Likelihood of this phenomenon increases with childbirth, age, and menopause.

Based on the above, we can see that normal continence requires that:

- abdominal pressure be transferred normally to the urethra;
- tonus of the sphincter be sufficient;
- perineum be elastic and have good tone;
- normal relationships between the organs be maintained;
- all pelvic tissues maintain normal mobility and elasticity.

## PATHOGENESIS OF INCONTINENCE

According to Beck (1965), over 50% of women experience stress incontinence during their first pregnancy. The problem often resolves without treatment. Pregnancy is the primary risk factor for incontinence.

With repeated childbirths, particularly with births involving forceps or suction, pelvic muscles and ligaments are stretched past their physiological limits. Fibers which are torn may be unable to recover healthy tonicity and elasticity. Large episiotomies, although sometimes necessary, lead to replacement of tissue with good tone and mobility by inelastic, non-mobile scar tissue. Pregnancy-related trauma may result in loss of elasticity of the anterior suspension of the urethra/bladder junction (type A incontinence). The anterior aspect of the bladder neck, which is attached to the pubic symphysis, is less affected by fetal motion than is the posterior aspect. Traumatic effects on the posterior aspect lead to hypotonia of the anchorage at the posterior symphysis by slackening the levators, particularly the expansion of the pubic portion of the levator ani behind the urethra/bladder junction.

Injuries which provoke incontinence include:

- injury to the levator ani;
- rupture of the tendinous arch of the pelvic fascia;
- distention or tearing of the vesicovaginal septum;
- distention or fibrosis of the pubovesical and pubo-urethral ligaments;
- ligamentous sacrococcygeal restrictions (caused by fetal motion or certain types of trauma);
- tiny restrictions of the trigone, bladder neck, or proximal urethra;
- bladder irritability;
- bladder/urethral inflammation (from diverse infectious agents);
- postpartum depression;
- sclerosis or secondary fibrosis after surgery;
- intrapelvic visceral ptoses or prolapses;
- intrapelvic visceral loss of mobility;
- certain rare neurological lesions (e.g., anterior branch of the pudendal nerve);
- articular lumbar/pelvic restrictions.

Essentially all lumbosacral traumas or restrictions adversely affect pelvic tonicity and sphincter control. In some cases, we have obtained good results through simple manipulation of the vertebral column. Given the extreme complexity of urogenital system innervation, it is no surprise that the exact mechanism of our therapeutic effects cannot always be explained.

Many urologists deny an association between incontinence and prolapse. While such association may not be universal, we know from experience that incontinence is very common in women with ptoses. "Prolapse" signifies that the contiguity of an organ's attachments has been lost. Varying degrees of ptosis (drooping) may occur before full prolapse. With most cases of secondary incontinence one finds a ptosis, though it may be minor. Some women do not consider the fact that they regularly lose a small amount of urine with effort "incontinence." However, these small losses are typical of those seen with a ptosis.

Factors other than injury or trauma which predispose to incontinence include:

- age (because of decreased tone and elasticity of muscles and connective tissue, vascular problems, kyphosis, etc.);
- obesity, pregnancy, tumors, or any increase of abdominal/pelvic pressure;
- chronic bronchitis, asthma, or other lung problems (because of the effect of coughing on pelvic structures);
- certain work-related postures and actions which provoke or aggravate incontinence;

- hormonal effects or interactions;
- medications (many anxiolytics and antidepressants impair bladder control, particularly in the male, and incontinence is often seen following anesthesia).

The stage of the menstrual cycle affects the degree of continency. The premenstrual period is the time of greatest risk because of increased uterine weight, altered orientation of genital organs, and diminishing urethral resistance. This latter effect may be due to the action of progesterone.

Menopause and related phenomena increase the incidence or degree of incontinence. Decreased estrogen levels after menopause are associated with the following phenomena (the mechanism is unknown in some cases):

- decreased density of connective tissue (particularly elastic fibers);
- decreased fluid content of tissues;
- hypotonia of sphincters;
- decreased reciprocal pressures of pelvic organs;
- diminished pressures in the cardiovascular system;
- general hypotonia;
- degeneration of lumbar/pelvic articulations;
- hypersensitivity of muscular mechanoreceptors.

## Bladder Hypersensitivity

Hyperstimulation of volume receptors or baroreceptors, or other abnormal stimuli, sometimes leads to incontinence. These factors occur, for example, with vesico-urethritis or urethrocystotrigonitis. They typically produce bladder instability with a feeling of urgency to urinate, rather than actual incontinence. The bladder instability can eventually lead to urethral instability.

## Alterations in Local Structure

Abnormal muscular/ligamentous pressures can provoke nociceptive stimuli and abnormally frequent urination (also known as pollakiuria). A urethrocystocele can irritate the trigonal region, which is particularly reflexogenic. Certain ptoses and prolapses compress and abnormally stimulate the trigonal/neck region. Similar problems are seen with bladder/vaginal sclerosis, and with adhesions secondary to trauma, childbirth, surgery, or radiation therapy.

## Hormonal Imbalance

The trigone and vagina share a common embryological origin and migration, and are both very hormone-dependent. As mentioned above, some types of incontinence are accentuated during the premenstrual period and improve just after the period begins. This has been attributed to progesterone deficiency and/or excessive estrogen. During pregnancy, abnormally frequent urination and nocturia are common. These symptoms usually appear long before the fetus is large enough to put pressure on the bladder, indicating that the cause is hormonal. The hormonal system also has a very strong effect on the venous plexuses in the bladder area. These (especially the plexus surrounding the bladder neck/urethra junction) play an important role in maintaining continence.

## Bladder Hypertonia

With abnormally high bladder tonus, the volume receptors and baroreceptors become hypersensitive. The subject may feel a need to urinate when there is less than 150ml of urine present (with a pressure of about 80cm $H_2O$). Possible causes include a history of bladder probes, fibrosis of the detrusor, and direct or indirect compressions of the bladder (e.g., from a tumor or retroverted uterus). Patients with hypersensitive bladders often also have enuresis. In our experience these are signs of relative immaturity of the central nervous system or a psychological dysfunction, often related to the family. The strong psychological repercussions frequently observed in cases of bladder irritability demonstrate the involvement of the nervous system in this problem.

## Lower Back Problems

Because of efferent stimulation from the spinal cord, chronic and debilitating lower back pain can cause or aggravate a hypersensitive bladder up to a state of irritability. Many patients pass from stress incontinence to total incontinence following a laminectomy. This may be partly explained by subdural fibrosis, which often occurs after this type of surgery. Impotence can also occur after lumbar surgery. As spinal blocks can lead to similar harmful effects on the meninges, we are wary of them.

## Neurological conditions

In stress incontinence, the patient remains continent unless there is some unusual stress on the bladder. In neurological incontinence, voluntary control of urination is not possible; urination is controlled solely by the autonomic nervous system. This condition is found with such illnesses as multiple sclerosis, cerebral tumor, atheroma, spina bifida, and advanced Parkinson's disease. Conditions such as diabetic neuropathy, chronic anemia, and thyrotoxicosis can also impair nervous control of the bladder function.

## Conclusion

Accurate differential diagnosis of incontinence before beginning any treatment is essential. Results are quite different when treating, for example, a hypersensitive bladder versus a fibrotic bladder restriction. Our goals are to defibrose and tonify the tissues, to recreate or release pelvic visceral mobility, and, as always, to restore proper osteo-articular mobility.

# *Indications for Bladder Manipulation*

Stress incontinence itself is by far the most common bladder disorder. Almost any functional disorder of the bladder is an indication for manipulation of the bladder. The following are the most common conditions that can be helped by bladder manipulations. Note that some are related to incontinence.

## Postpartum Dysfunction

As we have mentioned, at least 40% of women will suffer from stress incontinence at some point in their life, and childbirth is often the precipitating factor. There are three mechanisms underlying postpartum incontinence:

- mechanical: abnormal distention or retraction of muscular or connective fibers supporting the bladder and urethra.
- hormonal: fluid absorption by tissues leads to greater distention. Postpartum imbalance of estrogen and progesterone levels obviously has an effect on pelvic muscles and ligaments, although the mechanism is not fully understood. For this reason, a woman should wait at least 6 months after childbirth before undertaking any strenuous exercise program.
- reflexive: the neuronal/hormonal reflexes involved may be central (e.g., hypothalamic-pituitary axis) or local (e.g., originating from the pelvic organs or the sacroiliac joint).

## Bladder Prolapse

This is common in postmenopausal women and results from the central hypotonia which lasts about two years after menopause. The trigone and bladder neck areas are very hormone-dependent, which partly explains incontinences which stop without apparent reason. The full bladder should be smooth, or, more exactly, not collapsed upon its folds. In some cases of hypotonia and bladder prolapse, small folds appear and upset normal urinary function. This appears to be due to a reflex between the mucosa and parietal levels of the bladder which results in compression and residual stasis.

## Visceral Fixations and Adhesions

The bladder can adhere to any of the organs or tissues which surround it. These adhesions can change the functional position of the bladder (e.g., rotate or sidebend it), leading to pressure imbalances and possible incontinence. Adhesions of the superior surface often result from:

- surgery of the abdomen or pelvic area;
- sequelae of infections such as peritonitis, appendicitis, and pelvic inflammatory disease;
- childbirth, abortion, or trauma to the lumbar/sacrococcygeal area;
- sequelae of infections of the vulval and anal openings, often related to sexually-transmitted diseases;
- peritoneal microinfections too small to be called peritonitis, but sufficient to cause adhesion of different peritoneal layers or disruption of normal pressure distributions.

It is quite uncommon to find an abdomen without small adhesions. These are typically ignored by conventional physicians. Finding them requires great tactile sensitivity. They nonetheless have great diagnostic import, from the osteopathic perspective.

## Lithiasis

Bladder stones can, eventually, become troublesome and require surgical intervention. In the interest of helping a patient avoid surgery, if you are adventurous you may wish to try removing a stone from the bladder via the urethra. Be aware, though, that the urethra is very narrow and this procedure can be very painful. We once read in Testut (1889) that he had successfully put one finger in the urethral canal, dilating it to a few centimeters. We have tried this, and twice have successfully removed bladder stones via the urethra. These patients would otherwise have undergone surgery because of serious bladder and kidney infections. We do not know whether our manipulations have any effect upon stone formation.

## Other Syndromes

CYSTITIS AND CYSTALGIA: Numerous pathological processes can be covered by these vague terms or the equally vague term urinary tract infection. These range from simple bladder inflammation to very pathological recurring infections. Bladder irritations may also have psychological, hormonal, bacterial, viral, parasitic, or mechanical origins. We have been interested to discover that cystitis often arises from non-mobile structures. When this is the case, osteopathic treatment can be very useful.

DYSPAREUNIA AND ANORGASMIA: These disorders are provoked by collapse or fibrosis of tissues in contact with the bladder neck region, vesicovaginal fascia, or inferior part of the uterovesical fascia. There is always a painful retropubic anterior vaginal prominence which, when prodded, provokes sensations of pain and a need to urinate. These almost always occur postpartum where there has been a "well-accompanied" medical delivery. During intercourse, the pain is mostly felt in the prone position, when the penis presses upon the vesicovaginal attachments.

SPHINCTER DEFICIENCIES: Manipulation of the bladder has an undeniable local effect, but also a reflexogenic effect. Stretching stimulates various receptors in the bladder wall, leading to stimulatory effects on the detrusor and internal and external sphincters. This approach is often helpful in cases of ureterovesical reflux and sphincter hypotonia.

RESIDUAL BLADDER: This condition is typical of hypotonic bladders. A residual amount of urine always remains in the bladder, even immediately after urination. There is a certain risk of infection.

RESTRICTIONS AND UTERINE MALPOSITIONING: The bladder and uterus are highly interdependent. You must always manipulate these two organs in conjunction with each other. Normal urogenital functioning is impossible if the uterus is anteverted and anteflexed or if its fasciae are restricted.

ENURESIS IN CHILDREN: There is often a psychological component in these cases. However, we have also obtained excellent results solely by working on restrictions of vertebral segments traditionally associated with urinary dysfunction (T7, L1, L2, sacrum, coccyx). Manipulation of the vertebral column seems more effective than that of the bladder itself in these cases.

PREMENSTRUAL SYNDROME: The variety of causes and symptoms here is bewildering. Each type of medicine has its own view of this problem. We have treated many patients with PMS but have difficulty offering any generalizations; each case seems unique. We have had better luck with local manipulation (spine, pelvis, intrapelvic organs) than distant manipulation. We have also had more success with nonvirgins since we can utilize internal as well as external approaches.

# *Diagnosis*

## HISTORY

The history-taking process must be in-depth, complete, and respectful, but avoid pointless modesty. The urogenital region is a common site of tumor formation and you must be very alert to possible warning signs.

In stress incontinence, loss of urine always occurs during some unusual stress: coughing, sneezing, muscular exertion, anything which increases bladder pressure and presses on the sphincters. *A bladder which loses urine when there is no local stress demands careful attention.* Look for causes such as tumors, neurological, or hormonal phenomena. Try to pinpoint the incident or event which precipitated the problem: childbirth, a muscular effort, tenacious lower back pain, pelvic or sacrococcygeal trauma, etc. Sometimes there is no apparent reason. In the case of hematuria or foul-smelling urine, other tests will be necessary: urinalysis, CBC, ultrasound, intravenous urography, cystography, etc. Don't hesitate to send your patient to a urologist. No one can know everything and there are problems that cannot be helped by osteopathy.

## BEHAVIOR IN INCONTINENCE AND CYSTALGIA

The incontinent patient tries to reinforce or substitute for tonus of the bladder and its supporting structures, primarily by contracting the perineum and pelvitrochanteric muscles. When the bladder is under great tension, she actively contracts the muscles of external rotation. When tension is less, she adopts a position of relative internal rotation. In this position, the anterior perineum contracts, the urogenital fissure narrows, the ischiococcygeal muscles and levator ani contract, and the coccyx moves toward the pubis. Voluntary perineal contraction increases urethral pressure without changing pelvic and bladder pressures.

If the incontinent patient tries to increase perivesical muscular tension, the cystalgic patient does exactly the opposite. As soon as a particular region becomes painful, the body changes its position so that the tension of the neighboring muscles is decreased. For this reason, the cystalgic patient holds the pubis posteriorly and the thighs in internal rotation.

## DIFFERENTIAL DIAGNOSIS

Always ask yourself whether osteopathic manipulation is likely to actually benefit your patient. Taking on a patient for whom manipulation is inappropriate or useless is a serious error. What effect could bladder manipulation have on an acute urinary tract infection? An infection with such pathogens as *Chlamydia* or *Trichomonas* can lead to infertility. With bacterial infections such as these, antibiotic therapy is obviously the best treatment. We strongly urge the reader to learn to recognize the following conditions through differential diagnosis:

- urinary tract infection;
- polyp at the bladder neck;
- bladder stone;
- chronic urinary retention;

- bladder irritability;
- spinal abnormality (e.g., spina bifida);
- neuropathy (e.g., tabes dorsalis);
- systemic illness (e.g., diabetes);
- cerebral condition (e.g., multiple sclerosis);
- tumors of the urogenital or intestinal systems;
- psychogenic problems.

Of course, this list is not all-inclusive. It is intended simply as a starting point. Remember that hematuria is not normal and urgently requires further check-up. It is also important to note that one of the first symptoms of multiple sclerosis can be a bladder problem.

# Palpation and Mobility Tests

Note: throughout this and subsequent chapters, the terms "superiorly" and "upward" will mean toward the head, regardless of the position of the patient. Likewise, "inferiorly" and "downward" will mean away from the head.

## EXTERNAL APPROACH

The small intestine and greater omentum tend to invade the pelvis because of their mobility and distensibility. For example, when the bladder is empty, the loops of the small intestine often invade the uterovesical pouch. Sometimes one can even find a loop of the small intestine in the rectouterine pouch, making a colpocele. These areas must be tested for potential ptoses or restrictions. An intestinal ptosis or restriction has considerable influence upon the static position and mobility of the bladder *(Illustration 2-9)*.

These structures can be tested in the supine position, with legs bent *(Illustration 2-10)*, or in the seated position. The movement consists of bringing the small intestine upward, toward the umbilicus, following the arc of an imaginary circle located inside the cecum and ascending colon, and on the descending and sigmoid colon.

Use your fingers to bring the small intestine and greater omentum toward the umbilicus as if along the spokes of a bicycle wheel. A fixed zone will be painful and demand greater traction. Therefore, paradoxically, the first test for the bladder is that for the greater omentum and small intestine. Pay attention to the cecum also, since appendectomies often have an indirect effect on the bladder.

## Median and Medial Umbilical Ligaments

SUPINE POSITION: Be alert for any rupture of the muscular or connective fibers between the umbilicus and suprapubic region. Certain intense efforts can cause small tears of the median and medial umbilical ligaments. Although neither of these ligaments plays a suspensory role for the bladder, a scar, adhesion, or rupture here can disturb the normal transmission of tension and pressure, thereby affecting the mobility and motility of the bladder.

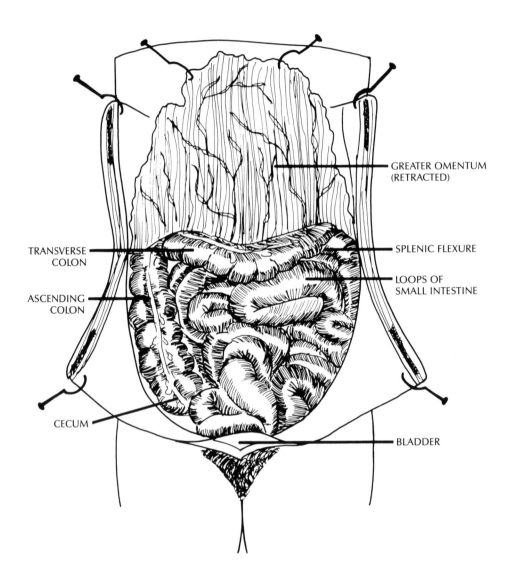

**Illustration 2-9**
Relationship between Bladder and Small Intestine

At different points along a line going from the umbilicus to the suprapubic region, pull the skin, subcutaneous adipose tissue, and rectus abdominis muscle toward you. Place your fingers between the halves of the rectus on the linea alba, or go from the lateral edge of the rectus toward the center. In patients with a separation of the rectus (which sometimes occurs during pregnancy), take advantage of this situation to get between the two medial edges of the rectus. You need to repeat this technique several times before you can be confident in distinguishing normal from abnormal tension of the median umbilical ligament. Where there is a restriction, you should feel a tension which is too great, and an irregular sliding of the tissues. Some patients have the impression of release during this technique.

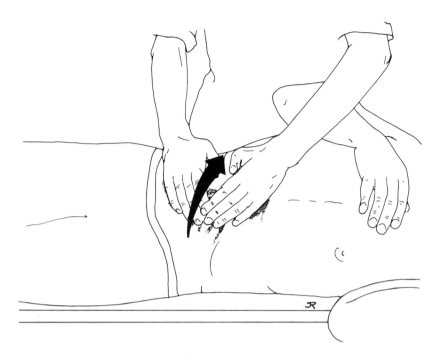

**Illustration 2-10**
Mobility Test of Small Intestine and Greater Omentum

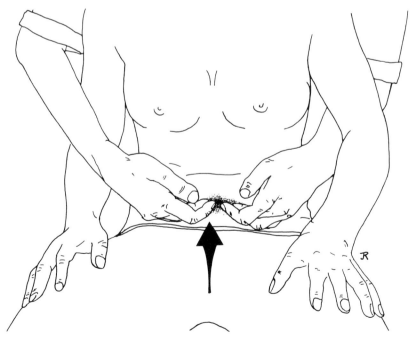

**Illustration 2-11**
Test of Median Umbilical Ligament

SEATED POSITION: We prefer this position because the effect of gravity is normal *(Illustration 2-11)*. Place your fingers on a line going from the umbilicus to the pubis; kyphose the patient in order to eliminate the tension of the abdominal muscles; only then, bring your fingers upward. The more the subject is kyphosed, the easier it will be to gently place your fingers deep into the abdomen. You do not need to press too far because these ligaments are just behind the rectus muscle.

For the medial umbilical ligaments, add a rotational component to your test. Place your fingers approximately two fingers lateral to the midline above the pubis and move them superiorly, posteriorly, and then to the left or right, depending upon which ligament is being tested. A restriction of the ligament will demand a stronger digital traction and decrease the rotation.

## Pubic Symphysis

Restriction of this articulation can, via the pubovesical ligaments, disturb the physiological anteroposterior movement of the bladder. We shall describe one test that recreates the complex mobility of the pubic symphysis. Most other tests of this structure focus on position or alignment.

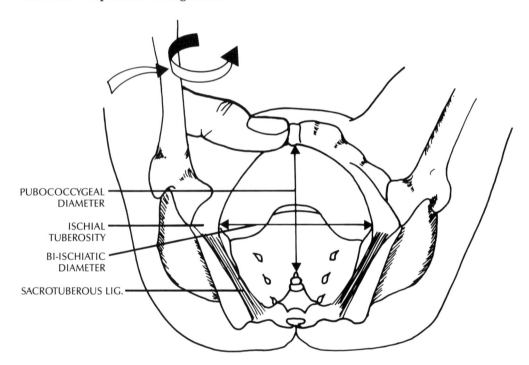

PUBOCOCCYGEAL DIAMETER

ISCHIAL TUBEROSITY

BI-ISCHIATIC DIAMETER

SACROTUBEROUS LIG.

**Illustration 2-12**
Test of Pubic Symphysis

The patient is supine and the leg on the side to be tested is bent. Place your thumb on the iliopubic ramus so that the pad is on the midline at the pubic symphysis. Mobilize the hip joint using combined movements in order to passively bring into play the pubic symphysis. With adduction and internal rotation, the tested iliopubic ramus will move closer to the table top, giving the impression that your fingers are moving downward. With abduction and external rotation, the iliopubic ramus moves upward and pushes against the fingers *(Illustration 2-12)*. Positional tests of the pubic symphysis are often misleading because of unequal development of the iliopubic rami, or because the bent leg is larger.

## Pubovesical Ligaments

SEATED POSITION:  These ligaments are tested in combination with the anterior vesical fascia. Place the fingers 2cm on either side of the linea alba and move them along the inferior lateral edges of the rectus abdominis. Kyphose the patient well in order to relax the inferior abdominal attachments. Your fingers will be on the medial part of the external orifice of the inguinal canal. Push the fingers posteriorly and then relax. Continue with small repetitive movements while looking for adhesions, areas of hypomobility, or scarring *(Illustration 2-13)*. For beginners, it is difficult to recognize restrictions in this area. As you are testing bilaterally, you can compare one side to the other.

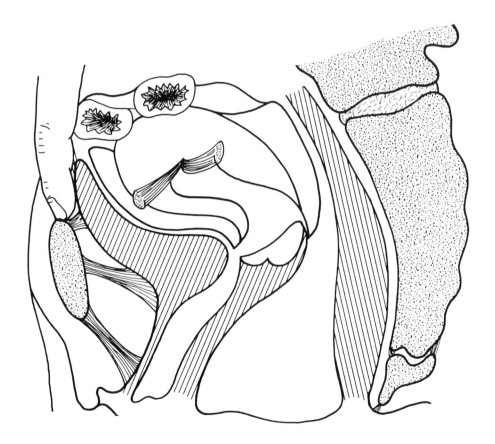

**Illustration 2-13**
Test of Pubovesical Ligaments: Seated Position

SUPINE POSITION: With the patient's legs bent, test with one hand the area behind the symphysis; with the other, flex the thighs up onto the abdomen to the degree allowed by the tension of the abdominal wall. Your fingers placed upon the medial part of the external inguinal canal go from lateral to medial, back to front, and top to bottom (Illustration 2-14).

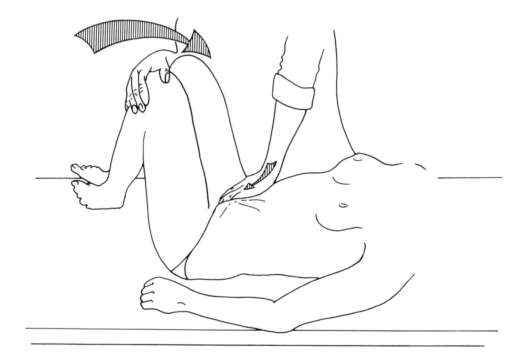

**Illustration 2-14**
Test of Pubovesical Ligaments: Supine Position

LATERAL DECUBITUS POSITION: Stand behind the patient, one hand testing the region behind the symphysis while the other mobilizes the thighs with flexion onto the trunk. The more the hips are flexed, the more deeply the fingers can explore the region to be tested. This position is comfortable for both patient and therapist, so we use it often.

KNEE / ELBOW POSITION: This position has the advantage of giving a sensation of weight to the pelvic organs, which are less supported by diaphragmatic attraction. Apart from contraction of the transversus, the abdominal muscles are not very tense and offer little resistance to movement of your fingers (Illustration 2-15). This position is also excellent for manipulation of the bladder.

STANDING POSITION: The patient stands, leaning forward, forearms on the table and head resting on the hands. Place your fingers first upon the median umbilical ligament and then upon the medial umbilical ligaments, and estimate their elasticity by pulling on each successively (Illustration 2-16). This position makes it easy to test the deep supravesical attachments.

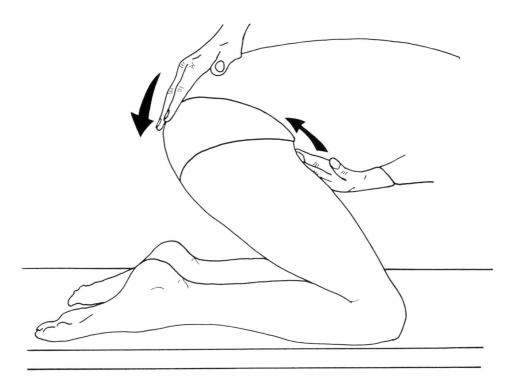

**Illustration 2-15**
Test of Pubovesical Ligaments: Knee/Elbow Position

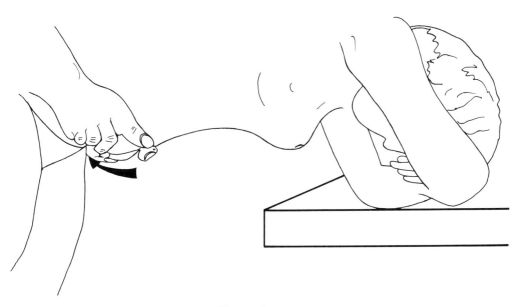

**Illustration 2-16**
Test of Pubovesical Ligaments: Standing Position

MODIFIED TRENDELENBURG POSITION:[1] You sit behind the table. The patient's sacrum and feet are on the table, her head and back resting on your thighs *(Illustration 2-17)*. An adjustable table will allow you to regulate the patient's slope and height. Use both hands to explore the region behind the symphysis; alternatively, use one hand to probe more deeply, while using the other to increase the flexion of the hips. You can also place one of the patient's feet upon the opposite thigh. This position may seem strange to the patient, but it does allow effective release of the tissues.

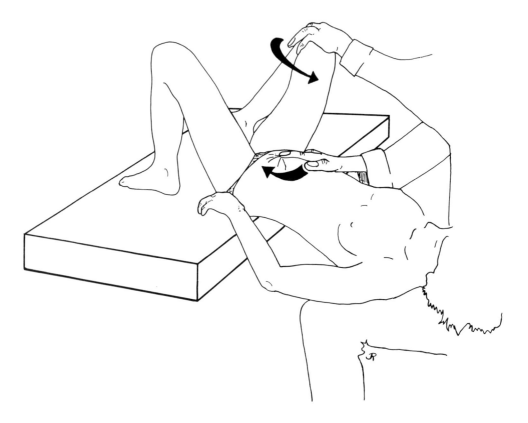

**Illustration 2-17**
Test of Pubovesical Ligaments: Modified Trendelenburg Position

In an alternative method, the patient puts her shoulders on the ground. Her pelvis rests upon a chair with the legs pressing against the back of the chair. Subsequent procedure is the same as above. We prefer the former method, but this one does allow the patient to treat herself at home.

1. Trendelenburg's position originally referred to the position of a patient on the operating table. As this modification (where the patient usually only has one part of his body on the table) was developed by Pierre Mercier, it is also known in France as "Mercier's declivious position." However we have used the term "Trendelenburg's position" or "Modified Trendelenburg position" throughout this book. Please note that in our earlier English books, we used the term "reverse Trendelenburg's position" for this same position.

## Perineal Body

During bladder testing, you must also evaluate the various components of the perineum. The perineal body, located between the vulva and anus, acts as the central nucleus for this region. To test the perineal body, place the patient in supine position and push the hard mass of the body superiorly *(Illustration 2-18)*. If the body is too easy to mobilize, or gives the impression of being flat and diffuse, you are dealing with a hypotonic and distended perineum. The perineal body is composed by interlacing of the muscular fibers of the levator ani, voluntary anal sphincter, vaginal constrictor muscles, and superficial and deep transverse perineal muscles. It can also be tested via the rectal or vaginal route, as described later.

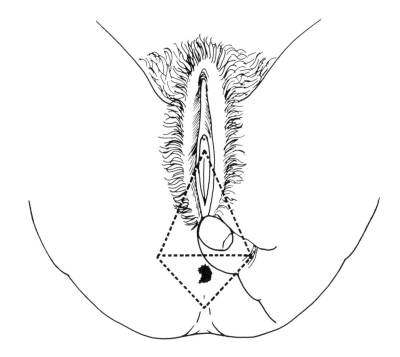

**Illustration 2-18**
Test of Perineal Body

## Obturator Foramina

These foramina have a close relationship with the bladder. The umbilicoprevesical aponeurosis rests against the median umbilical ligament, and the umbilical arteries rest against the anterior parietal peritoneum. The aponeurosis continues as the prevesical fascia which surrounds the anterior and lateral sides of the bladder. The fascia then follows the pubovesical ligaments which, laterally, fuse with the pelvic aponeurosis until the sciatic anchorage points. It rejoins the internal obturator muscle, levator ani, and, above all, the aponeuroses. With bladder problems (especially bacterial infection), we frequently observe fibrosis of tissues in or around the obturator foramen.

The foramina are tested with the patient in supine position, the leg of the tested side flexed, and the other stretched out. With your hand open, slide the thumb along the adductors to the point of insertion of the adductor magnus and pectineus muscles *(Illustration 2-19)*. Try not to get your thumb stuck between the iliopubic and ischiopubic rami. If this happens, move laterally and posteriorly around them into the obturator foramen. We prefer to go through the obturator foramen because it is easier; there is more room and much less resistance by muscles and tendons. We have checked this technique with fluoroscopy. The thumb goes approximately 1cm inside the foramen in a patient of average weight and height, and even deeper in thin patients.

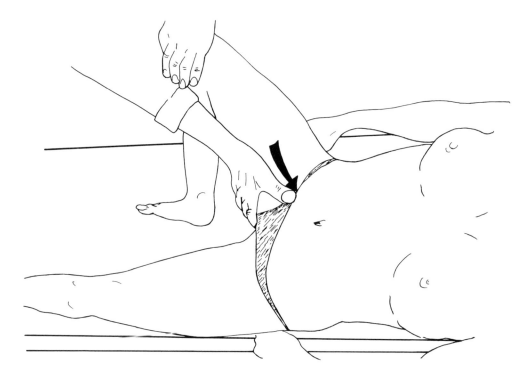

**Illustration 2-19**
Test of Obturator Foramen

When the thumb has gone as far as possible, test the surrounding tissues. Ask the patient to breathe in and out deeply (or cough). With practice, you will get the feeling of a membrane which stretches and relaxes with respiration. Strangely, with a significant restriction, you may feel the strongest push of the membrane during exhalation. Perhaps, in people who are not aware of respiratory problems, contraction of the abdominal muscles is used to increase intracavitary pelvic pressure at the end of exhalation.

With an internal restriction, your thumbs will feel stronger resistance. With ptosis, it will be easier to go deep into the foramen. Either one of these results should be considered abnormal. You must always compare both sides as often only one side is affected. In the healthy subject, both sides should offer the same resistance. During the test, the other fingers can evaluate the tissues of the ischiorectal region. One can carry out this test in the standing position, but there is a risk that the patient will be embarrassed.

In the same position, you can evaluate the ischiorectal region and anococcygeal body. Move your hand from the medial edge of the ischium toward the anus and perineal body. First stretch the tissues toward the anus and then bring them back toward the ischium.

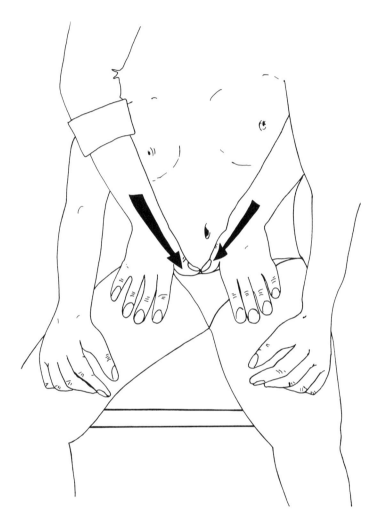

**Illustration 2-20**
Aggravation Test

## Aggravation Tests

The above tests are sometimes inconclusive. If you remain unsure of the condition of an attachment of the bladder, compress it downward instead of stretching it upward. If the patient has a restriction, she will experience transient incontinence or feel pain in a specific location. For example, suppose you have found abnormal tension in the right superior prevesical retropubic region. With the patient seated, compress the affected region and push gently downward *(Illustration 2-20)*. If the region has no restriction, the patient will feel neither tension nor the urge to urinate. Also, ask the patient to cough. If your fingers are exactly upon a pathogenic restriction, the pressure will seem unbearable and the patient will ask you to remove your fingers.

### Indirect Tests Using the Legs

As explained above, the bladder is closely related with the obturator foramen via fasciae, membranes, and muscles. Restrictions in and around this region can cause fibrosis of the pelvitrochanteric muscles, leading to restricted range of motion of the hip joint. Restrictions are most commonly found in the internal obturator and piriformis muscles, which affect the quadratus femoris and external obturator. When the patient perceives pain at a precise location in the hip joint during mobilization, mechanical problems of the bladder are indicated. This is due to fibers (known as the acetabular ligament) running from the hip joint to the internal obturator fascia and bladder. With degenerative joint disease, this ligament can pull the bladder laterally, and bladder discomfort can be provoked by lateral movement of the hip.

The internal obturator muscle arises from the periphery of the obturator foramen, and inserts on the greater trochanter of the femur. It causes external rotation and abduction of the thigh. If the thigh is internally rotated and adducted, the attachments of this muscle around the obturator will be put under tension and any associated visceral restriction will be stretched *(Illustration 2-21)*. This causes hypersensitivity of the bladder and an urge to urinate.

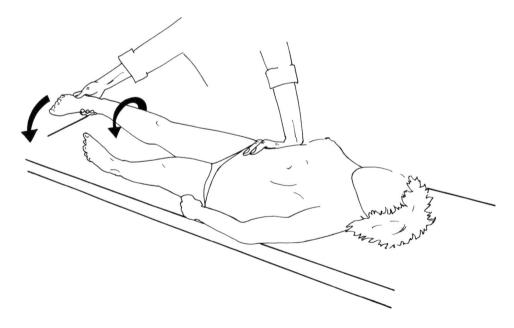

**Illustration 2-21**
Stretching the Internal Obturator Muscle

## INTERNAL APPROACH

The pubovesical ligaments are composed partly of muscular fasciculi arising from the external layer of the detrusor. This creates an elastic anchorage which enables the neck of the bladder to move posteroinferiorly. The trigonal/neck region is anchored to the pelvic floor and rests upon the anterior wall of the vagina. As mentioned earlier, the bladder has an anchorage system with two components: anterior (more active) and posterolateral (more passive) (see *Illustration 2-4*). These must always be evaluated in patients with bladder problems. Here, we will describe methods for testing these anchorage systems.

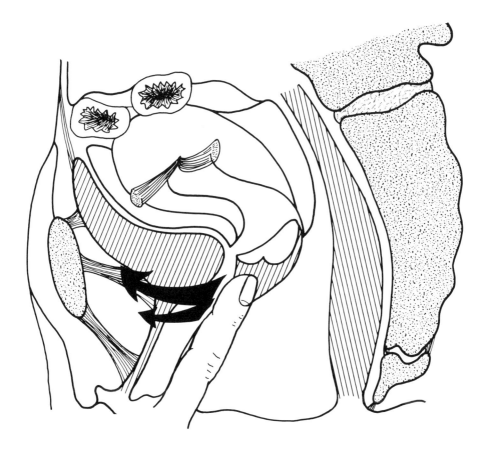

**Illustration 2-22**
Trigonal/Neck Test

## Trigonal/Neck Region

The patient is supine, legs slightly apart. In this same position, you can check the position of the cervix and to see if the uterus is low, retroflexed, anteflexed, etc. (see chapter 3). The status of the uterus can affect your treatment of the bladder. For example, if significant cervical restrictions exist, they must be treated before you can effectively work with the trigonal/neck region. Place the anterior surface of your index finger against the anterior vaginal wall and push it toward the inferior edge of the pubic symphysis (*Illustration 2-22*). The trigonal/neck region is felt as a thicker and slightly harder area, like a wet handkerchief. It is abnormal to feel it as soon as you try, as this means that it is too far down. Determine whether it protrudes toward the back, is low, or is easy to mobilize. A bladder prolapse can cause a cervicocystocele.

In the case of a significant restriction, mobilization can be painful and provoke an urge to urinate, or even slight incontinence. Pain is often due to an inflammation or infection of the trigonal/neck region. In the case of cystocervical ptosis with injury to the anterior anchorage system, but without cervicocystocele, you will have the impression of feeling a bud. This problem, often resulting from childbirth, is typically the basis of dyspareunia occurring when the woman is prone. The trigonal/neck region irritates the vesicovaginal fascia, which is an erogenous zone.

In the presence of a restriction or posteroinferior collapse of the trigonal/neck region, ask the patient to perform retention and pushing movements of the bladder. This will increase the information you can gain from these tests. During a *retention effort* the anterior anchorage system contracts, while the posterior system remains fixed. The urethral cap moves forward, so much so that the stretched trigonal/neck region is normally not felt under the fingers. If the trigonal/neck region continues to be perceptible, the anterior system is lax or even broken; another possibility is that the posterior system is fixed. During a *pushing effort* the anterior system relaxes and causes the urethral cap to disappear, and the trigonal/neck region moves posteriorly and pushes against your finger. If this displacement does not take place, the anterior system is fixed. Difficulty in return to the normal position indicates a partial posterior restriction.

To conclude: if the trigonal/neck region can always be felt under your finger, there is a significant restriction of the posterior anchorage system and a laxity of the anterior system. If with a pushing effort the trigonal/neck region cannot be felt, the anterior anchorage system is fixed. This is a problem with a better prognosis, as we shall see.

## Vesical Body

Use the conventional bimanual abdominal/vaginal exam. The abdominal hand palpates and mobilizes the bladder. The intravaginal fingers (usually two) push toward the abdominal hand in order to make the tissues slide upon one another (*Illustration 2-23*). The bladder can be tested in three planes:

- vertical plane: the intravaginal fingers are pushed, e.g., toward the anterior vaginal pouch, and serve as a fixed pressure point for the abdominal hand, which makes the tissues move from top to bottom.
- transverse plane: the abdominal hand causes the tissues to slide from side to side on top of the intravaginal fingers.
- frontal plane: the palm of the abdominal hand stretches the tissues in a circular manner on the intravaginal fingers, in a clockwise direction and then counterclockwise.

With this technique, you can detect folds, scars, adhesions, fibrosis, hypomobility, or hypermobility. Be cautious in reaching your diagnosis. An adhesion may only be palpable in one plane, and the hand can easily be misled.

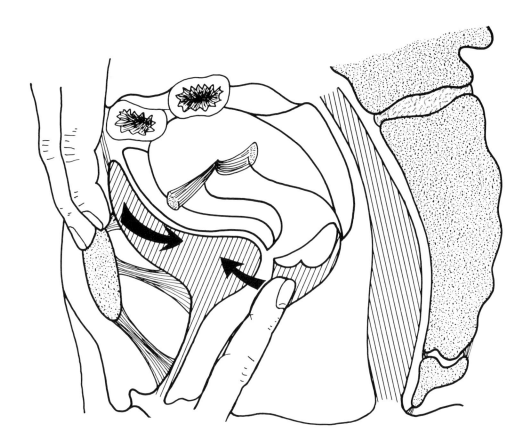

**Illustration 2-23**
Test of Vesical Body

## Urethral Stretching

Urethral pressure is modulated by smooth muscles, striated muscles, elastic attachments of the bladder neck, and the vascular plexus of the submucosa. You should know how to determine if the urethra can be stretched longitudinally. Artificial lengthening of the urethra provokes an increase of intraluminal pressure which may be as high as 40% according to Renaud (1980). With certain infectious or mechanical sequelae, the urethra remains stuck to the bladder neck, vaginal wall, or pubo-urethral ligaments. Urethral stretching is performed in the bimanual exam position, the intravaginal finger pressing against the posterior part of the pubis and stretching it anterosuperiorly *(Illustration 2-24)*. The abdominal fingers, in the suprapubic position, also indirectly pull the urethral and periurethral structures superiorly. This test is positive if the stretched structures cannot be distended, if they are sensitive, or if you feel a little bump which signifies fibrosis around part of the urethra.

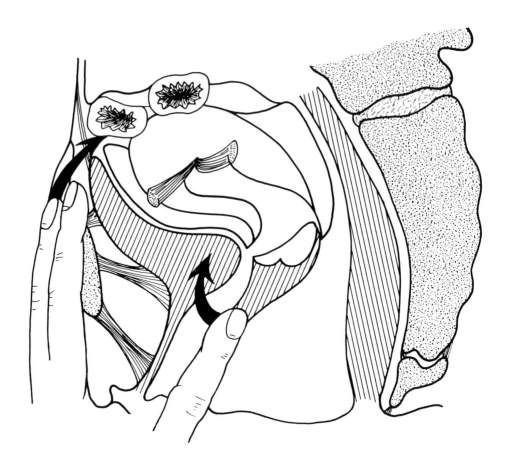

**Illustration 2-24**
Urethral Stretching

### Levator Ani

The fasciculi of the sphincter ani are bilaterally palpated by two intravaginal fingers separated slightly and directed laterally toward the ischial fossae *(Illustration 2-25)*. When the patient makes a retention effort, you will feel two stretched cords; evaluate their tonicity. With more aged or lax patients, test one fascicula at a time.

There are fasciculi found on the most anterior part of the pelvic floor, just above the vulva. With your forearms between the patient's legs, ask her to carry out an opposing active adduction by tightly holding your arm or shoulder tightly. Where she pushes will depend upon the length of the upper limb of the practitioner and the length of the lower limbs of the patient. Evaluate for excessive tightness or laxity.

### Uterosacral Ligaments and Parametrium

The two intravaginal fingers push laterally on the lateral pouches of the cervix *(Illustration 2-26)*. Pain provoked by this test could be due to partial rupture of the

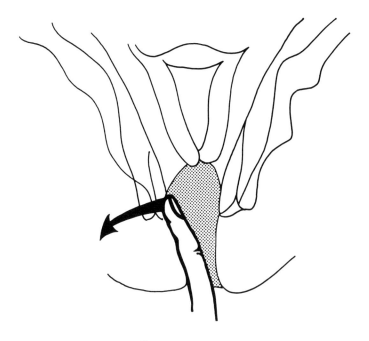

**Illustration 2-25**
Test of Fasciculi of Sphincter Ani

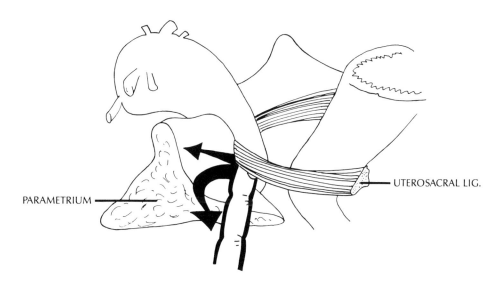

PARAMETRIUM

UTEROSACRAL LIG.

**Illustration 2-26**
Test of Uterosacral Ligaments and Parametrium

uterosacral ligaments, which often causes the cervix to move toward the side of the problem because of retracted and fibrosed tissues. With complete rupture of the ligament, the cervix moves toward the contralateral side because the tonicity of the opposing tissues is lost. With bilateral complete rupture, the cervix collapses forward and the body of the uterus toward the back. Chapter 3 includes a description of Masters and Allen syndrome, caused by rupture of the uterosacral ligaments after a difficult childbirth.

### Rectovaginal Exam

The rectovaginal exam is performed with one finger in the vagina and another intrarectal. This exam can be used to evaluate the thickness and consistency of the perineal body and rectovaginal septum. The cervix should be neither too readily apparent nor too difficult to push away. If upon pushing you get the impression of an omentum or loop of the small intestine under the two fingers, you may be feeling a colpocele. This test is seldom used because it is uncomfortable for the patient and usually does not give any more information than a regular vaginal exam.

Internal (rectal or vaginal) testing should not be routinely used unless prior external (abdominal) tests were positive. In some cases (e.g., incontinence or dyspareunia), however, internal tests are more likely to give useful information.

## COCCYX

As mentioned earlier, coccygeal restrictions have a great influence on bladder function. In fact, we would say that *it is almost impossible to achieve positive effects through manipulation of the bladder if the coccyx is fixed.* Tests of the coccyx are not well known and often neglected when they are known. We urge you to familiarize yourself with the following tests of the coccyx.

A coccygeal restriction can be of direct articular origin (e.g., restriction of the sacrococcygeal joint with retraction of the anterior or posterior sacrococcygeal ligaments) or of indirect origin (e.g., problems of the posterolateral anchorage system which involves the uterosacral ligaments, parametrium, coccygeus muscles, some fibers of the piriformis, internal obturator, small and large sacrotuberous ligaments, and anococcygeal body). These restrictions are often unilateral, and require a sound knowledge of tests in the sidebending position.

For the following three external tests, start with the patient seated on the table, legs slightly apart and dangling. Have her place her weight on one ischial tuberosity. Place your index and middle fingers far in front of the coccyx. Note that beginners never put their fingers far enough forward, and end up on the sacrum instead of the coccyx. To do this properly, put your fingers as far forward as possible and then bring them back slightly if necessary. Have the patient put her weight on one tuberosity and then the other. Then have her bend slightly forward. This procedure separates the tuberosities and stretches the tissues which insert on them.

### Anterior-Posterior Test

Push the coccyx superiorly and slightly anteriorly *(Illustration 2-27)*, then move it inferiorly and slightly posteriorly. If there is a restriction, this movement will be very painful or even unbearable. Anterior restrictions (which are more common) usually result from direct trauma to the area. Posterior restrictions are often due to a difficult childbirth.

### Lateral Flexion Test

With the fingers of one hand on the coccyx, sidebend the patient (by her shoulders) to each side in turn. Normally the coccyx will slide to the ipsilateral side. When

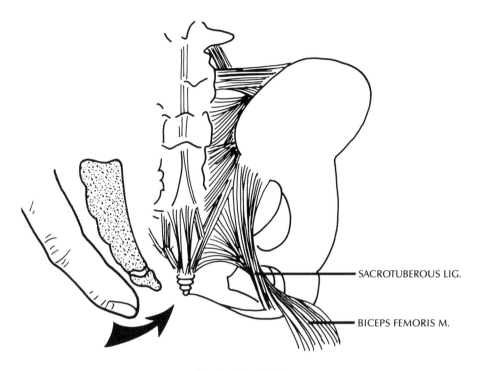

**Illustration 2-27**
Anterior-Posterior Coccygeal Test

the coccyx slides in only one direction but remains solidly connected to the ischium on one side, there is a restriction on that side.

Alternatively, use one hand to hold the ischium in place, and move the sacrum and coccyx away from the ischium with the other hand. As this is happening, evaluate the elasticity of the sacrotuberous and sacrospinous ligaments, which is more important than the degree of gross movement present. It may be helpful to compress the area before separation.

The sacrotuberous ligaments are always tight when the patient is seated. For many patients you will get clearer results if you test them with the patient supine. Put your finger on one side of the coccyx and push it toward the opposite side. Often there is greater tension on one side than the other. This may indicate a problem with a pelvic organ on that side.

## Bent-Knee Test

The patient stands with both hands against a wall, one leg (on the side of the sacrococcygeal restriction) bent and the other extended. For this example, assume that the restriction is on the left side. The patient flexes and extends the left thigh. Place your right thumb underneath the sacrococcygeal joint and your left thumb upon the ischium of the left leg. When the thigh flexes, the left ischium moves anterosuperiorly *(Illustration 2-28)*. If there is a restriction, particularly of the sacrospinous or sacrotuberous ligament, the ischium moves only very slightly, and the sacrum compensates by sidebending.

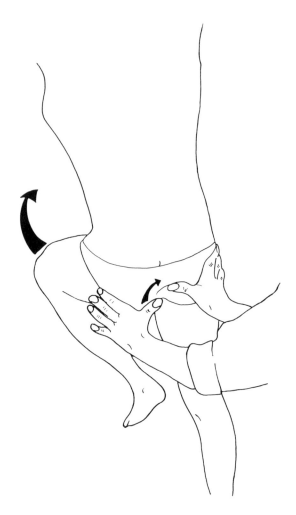

**Illustration 2-28**
Bent-Knee Test of Sacrococcygeal Ligaments


To simultaneously test the piriformis and internal and external obturators, have the patient perform active external rotation and abduction of the hip. We prefer that in testing the posterior muscles, the motion be generated by anterior muscles. This allows a better appreciation of the motion, especially when adduction is added to stretch the muscular fibers. Always compare both sides.

It is difficult to selectively pinpoint a muscle or ligament as the "real" problem. Consider the coccygeus muscle. It can be said to continue below the piriformis by inserting itself upon the coccyx, sciatic spine, deep surface of the sacrospinous ligament, and part of the aponeurosis of the internal obturator! Thus, it is hard to differentiate restrictions of the ischiococcygeal muscles versus the sacrococcygeal ligaments. Nevertheless, if you detect any restriction of movement or lack of elasticity, you must be as precise as possible in order to design an effective technique.

## Rectal Test

Place your index finger in the rectum with the pad of the tip on the sacrum and the rest of the finger against the coccyx. Your thumb is placed externally on the coccyx. With the other hand, compress the sacrum and flex the coccyx anteriorly-posteriorly *(Illustration 2-29)*. Normally there is approximately 30° of movement. Two types of restriction can be diagnosed:

- if the anterior sacrococcygeal ligaments are injured (due to direct trauma), the coccyx remains fixed anteriorly, and can be flexed but is difficult or impossible to bring into extension;
- if the posterior sacrococcygeal ligaments are fixed (because of difficult childbirth), the coccyx cannot flex anteriorly, but can be extended several degrees.

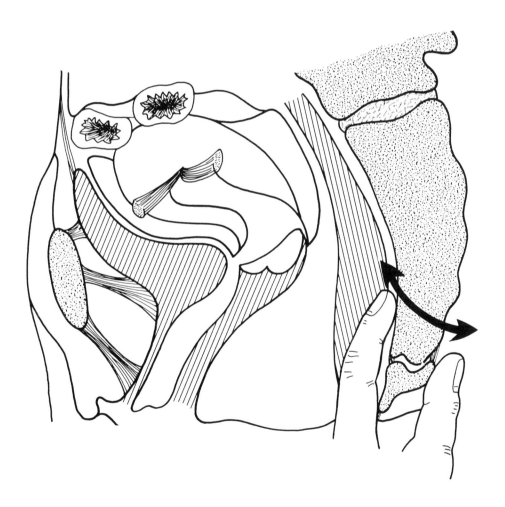

**Illustration 2-29**
Rectal Test of Sacrococcygeal Articulation

## ADVICE

The tests relating to bladder mobility and function which have been presented here have been evaluated clinically, by radiography, and by ultrasound wherever possible. Of course, you do not need to carry out all these tests for the sake of completeness. Follow a vertical testing hierarchy: a simple, positive test should be followed by another, more elaborate test, and so forth. We emphasize again that the patient is a whole, integrated organism in which all the parts are interrelated. Legs with varicose veins are a sign of insufficient venous return through the pelvis. The bladder and uterus, if too heavy, pull on their ligaments which, in turn, fibrose.

Aside from mechanical manipulation, you should inquire about the patient's lifestyle and diet. Pelvic function is affected by how a person spends most of the day. People who work in a standing position will tend to develop restrictions and venous congestion more in the anterior part of the pelvis (pubovesical ligaments, umbilical ligaments, trigone, etc.) People with desk jobs will tend to have posterior (uterosacral, sacrococcygeal, etc.) problems. A patient who sits all day should be advised to raise her legs for a while after getting home.

Diet is, as usual, a complex subject. There are two important guidelines: (1) patients with bladder problems should drink often, but not much at a time (to avoid overloading the bladder; and (2) they should avoid certain foods (e.g., asparagus, radishes, cabbage) which irritate the bladder and worsen the odor associated with incontinence.

# *Motility*

## SACROPELVIC MOTILITY TEST

The motions of motility for the bladder are the same as for the uterus, probably because of the common embryological origin of these organs. The expir phase of bladder motility consists of an anteroposterior movement, accompanied by a slight superior ascending component. For the sacropelvic test, place the heel of your palm on the suprapubic region with the fingers pointing toward the umbilicus. During expir, you should feel the palm move posterosuperiorly toward the umbilicus (*Illustration 2-30*).

This test is best performed with the patient in supine position, one of your hands over the suprapubic region, and the other under the sacrum. Place the palm of the sacral hand at the level of S2-S3 and the ends of the fingers on L5-S1. During expir, the heel of the sacral hand moves anteroinferiorly while the abdominal hand moves posterosuperiorly. Movement is abnormal if the hands are drawn in any other direction. This motion of the sacropelvic area should not be confused with that of the cranial rhythmic impulse (CRI). Some practitioners tend to force the sacrum to follow the rhythm of the bladder.

A combination of motility testing and local listening is very helpful when evaluating patients with bladder dysfunction. For example, what would you feel in a patient with a high uterovesical restriction? During the expir phase of motility, your abdominal hand would move superiorly but not posteriorly. Doing local listening, the palm of your hand would be attracted to the same place. If inhibition was applied to this area and motility rechecked, it would (temporarily) become normal.

A restriction, regardless of type or location, always attracts the practitioner's hand. We have verified this hundreds of times with dressed patients about whom we knew

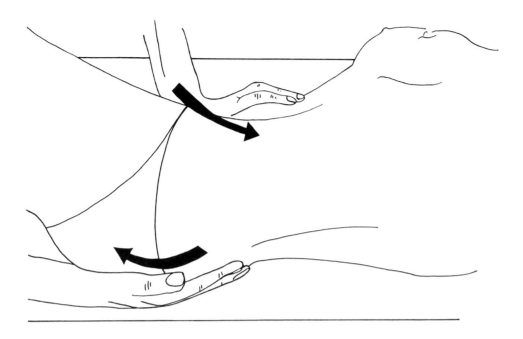

**Illustration 2-30**
Sacropelvic Motility Test: Expir

nothing. This phenomenon allows us to determine the position and sometimes even the nature of the restriction. Experienced osteopaths rely mainly on listening techniques to localize problems, and, if necessary, use internal exams for corroboration.

# *Restrictions*

Restrictions occur when tissues suffer an injury to their distensibility, mobility, or motility. Such injuries can result in either impairment or total absence of movement (both mobility and motility).

## SMALL INTESTINE, GREATER OMENTUM, PERITONEUM

The small intestine and associated structures affect the bladder in numerous ways. After enteritis, the small intestine and mesentery may be fixed, usually inferiorly. The small intestine therefore presses too hard against the bladder. Under normal conditions, it presses against it enough to leave small impressions, but remains sufficiently mobile to follow the diaphragmatic movements and pass them on. If it presses too hard, it can disrupt mechanical function of the bladder.

Most septic injuries to the small intestine are accompanied by peritoneal adhesions. Every movement of the body (respiration, walking, running, or whatever) disturbs the intestinal/bladder axis, and the peritoneum can no longer serve as a link between the diaphragm and abdominal/pelvic structures. The superior attraction of the diaphragm is decreased or even lost. If pressure of the intestine upon the bladder is chronically high, risk of incontinence is increased, anteroposterior mobility diminishes, or the bladder may be immobilized in a posteroinferior position.

## PUBIS

Pubic restrictions usually result from injuries to the interosseous or anterior ligaments, e.g., during childbirth or trauma indirectly transmitted by the lower limbs. The most common cause is an unexpected movement which transfers abrupt tensions to the pubic rami, as when you miss a stair.

## MEDIAN AND MEDIAL UMBILICAL LIGAMENTS

These ligaments are commonly injured during abdominal/pelvic surgery. They can be separated by median abdominal incisions. Sutures and scarring retract the fibers and modify their tension. The median and medial umbilical ligaments have a role in "suspensory tension." Damage to them prevents normal anteroposterior movement, and the bladder no longer moves posteroinferiorly, but remains "suspended." On local listening the hand is drawn superiorly and slightly anteriorly. A satisfactory structural environment for an organ requires that the membranous tensions surrounding it are well balanced. Disturbance of a single component affects the overall balance and can have widespread visceral effects.

## PUBOVESICAL AND PUBO-URETHRAL LIGAMENTS

These ligaments can be injured by obstetrical trauma, chronic cystitis or urethritis, or scarring. Restriction of these ligaments often leads to type A stress incontinence (see earlier section). This type of incontinence involves loss of elasticity of the anterior suspensions of the urethra/bladder junction and chronic opening of the bladder neck. The bladder remains pressed against the pubis with effort, instead of moving away. The neck of the bladder opens and lets urine out because the anterior edge stays with the pubis, while the posterior edge moves posteroinferiorly. Release of the anterior structures improves continence in a lasting manner.

## BLADDER SUPPORT

When it expels urine, the bladder moves posteriorly and descends so that it rests upon the cervix and vagina. This support system can be damaged by fibrosis or collapse; the latter condition, unfortunately, is more common and more difficult to treat. Injuries to muscles and ligaments in this area also affect the levator ani, uterosacral ligaments, coccygeus, obturators, piriformis, and superficial transverse perineal muscles. They are associated with perineal obstetrical tears or traumas, unsuccessful sutures of the perineum, or large episiotomies.

When bladder support is too weak, the bladder collapses upon the cervix and vagina, which collapse in turn. The bladder is locked in a pushing position, which promotes incontinence.

If bladder support is hard and fibrotic, the bladder can no longer move postero-inferiorly but stays fixed in a retention position, increasing the likelihood of a residual bladder. We have had better results with cases of fibrosis and lack of elasticity than with those of ruptures and significant weakness.

## UTERUS

The bladder, uterus, and rectum are physically and functionally related. Incontinence, cystitis, or cystalgia are often due to uterine malpositioning of three types:

- uterine anteversion and anteflexion: the body and to a lesser extent the cervix press hard against the bladder, increasing bladder pressure at the expense of sphincter pressure;
- uterine retroversion with anteflexion: irritates the trigonal/ bladder neck region and impairs continence;
- uterine prolapse: this can lead to prolapse of the bladder neck region.

A simple uterine verticalization modifies bladder pressure and mobility. In chapter 3 we shall discuss pathogenic aspects of uterus/bladder relationships in more detail, focusing on the cervix.

# *Manipulations*

## GOALS OF MANIPULATION

Our first goal is to return the mobility of partially or totally restricted structures. As soon as the bladder has recovered normal motion, integrate it into the global movement of the body and harmonize its motion with that of the other organs. In osteopathy, we always go from the specific to the general: from the cell to the tissue, tissue to organ, organ to function, and from specific function to general homeostasis. Isolated manipulations are pointless in our treatment philosophy.

The following are primary aims of urogenital visceral manipulation:

- release the tissues from restrictions
- restore normal physiology
- promote fluid circulation (arterial, venous, lymphatic, and interstitial)
- reduce inflammation and pain
- reinforce tonus of the abdominal wall
- reinforce the occlusive functions of sphincters
- ensure proper function of local and central nervous system
- stimulate local and central hormonal functions
- optimize transmission and distribution of abdominal/pelvic pressures
- aid in evacuation of stones
- enhance overall mind/body energy and well-being.

## CONTRAINDICATIONS

All direct techniques move tissues against other tissues, and therefore run some risk of creating inflammation, irritation, or microhemorrhage. Even when osteopathic manipulations are carried out very gently (as they should always be), the presence of a foreign body increases the risk of tissue injury through rubbing. For this reason, pregnancy, I.U.D.s, tumors, and stones are major contraindications to manipulation of urogenital structures.

Based on our experience, techniques that work on motility are not contraindicated during pregnancy or any other time.

### Pregnancy

Pregnancy is an absolute contraindication for internal work. Direct bladder manipulation always causes movement of the uterus and related structures. The fetus is so fragile and so important that it is foolish to take the chance of injuring it. Wait until after the birth of the child to attempt any direct manipulation of this area.

### I.U.D.s

Except for very experienced practitioners, no one should do internal work in the presence of an intrauterine device (I.U.D.) We have seen several cases of uterine bleeding when novices have ignored this advice. There is also the risk of dislodging the I.U.D. so that it becomes ineffective.

Interestingly, global and local listening easily reveal the presence of these devices even in fully clothed subjects. On listening, the hand is drawn toward anything which disturbs motility. It is very rare that an I.U.D., no matter how well placed, does not disturb the uterine mucosa.

### Tumors

Malignant or benign, a bleeding tumor is a contraindication for any direct technique because of the significant risk of increased hemorrhage. On the other hand, induction techniques are appropriate. Never imply to a patient that osteopathy can "cure" cancer. When we discover neoplastic tumors in our practice (which is relatively frequently) we send our patients as quickly as possible to cancer specialists. These patients often require conventional treatments such as chemotherapy or radiation.

If a member of your immediate family had a malignant tumor, would you treat him or her solely by manipulation? We hope not! We have heard some of our "colleagues" declare, decisively, that they have had "good results" with cancer. We wish they would tell us of the number of cases treated successfully by osteopathy (hopefully at least a hundred), so we can help spread the good word. If they are referring to vague, coincidental, or unexplained improvement in one or two patients, we wish they would just keep quiet!

When a patient has undergone radiation treatment for a pelvic tumor, the tissues often become very hard and even brittle. Mobility techniques should be used with extreme caution, or not at all, in these cases. Induction techniques can probably be used to promote homeostasis or energize an organ.

### Infections, Stones

Great care should be taken with acute bladder infections, especially pelvic inflammatory disease. In these cases, it is essential to precisely identify the pathogenic agent, and prescribe an antibiotic if appropriate. An untreated infection can easily lead to infertility.

It is sometimes wiser to leave a stone in the bottom of the bladder than try to force it out. If you try to force it, it may end up blocking the proximal urethral opening.

## EXTERNAL TECHNIQUES

### Small Intestine, Greater Omentum

Imagine that the umbilicus is the hub of a wheel and that the attachments of the small intestine are represented by the spokes of this wheel. This is an approximation of the roots of the mesentery, from the cecum to the duodenojejunal junction. The best

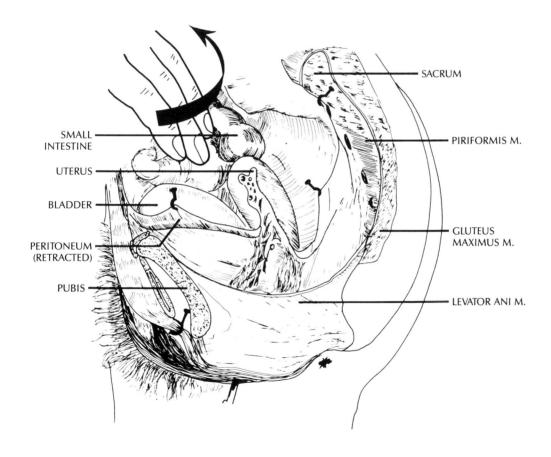

**Illustration 2-31**
Manipulation of Small Intestine

way to treat the small intestine is via the roots of the mesentery. Place your fingers inferior to the root, moving slowly posteriorly and then superiorly until you feel the root. Pull superiorly on the root in a rhythmic fashion. Keep your rhythm in tune with the tissues and focus on the areas that feel tight. Continue until you feel a release along the entire root (*Illustration 2-31*). These technique can be performed in the dorsal, lateral decubitus, or modified Trendelenburg position. See *Visceral Manipulation* (pp. 153-4) and *Visceral Manipulation II* (pp. 189-91) for more details.

### Pubic Symphysis

A commonly-used technique for dysfunctions of this area is to have the patient isometrically contract the adductors by squeezing her knees together. We have never found this to be particularly effective. Try the following technique instead. With the patient supine, place your shoeless foot gently upon the pubic symphysis on the side opposite the restriction. Hold on to the foot of the patient's extended lower leg with both hands, and vary the amount of hip flexion in order to focus on the restriction.

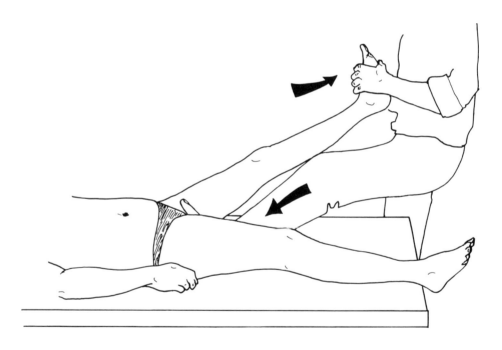

**Illustration 2-32**
Manipulation of Pubis

For example, if the iliopubic ramus is inferior (lower) on the right, stand on the patient's left. Glide your left foot along the adductors until your first metatarsophalangeal joint is on the right pubis. While your foot stabilizes the iliopubic ramus, focus the tension on the exact area of the restriction by using traction and (usually) internal rotation. Then perform a quick but gentle "thrust" using traction on the left leg, which is slightly off the table (*Illustration 2-32*). Many variations of this technique are possible.

## Median and Medial Umbilical Ligaments

SEATED POSITION:  Stand behind the patient, who is sitting on the table, legs slightly apart. Place your fingers on a line running from the umbilicus to the suprapubic region, facing the vesical apex. In the beginning the patient should be kyphosed, which relaxes the abdominal muscles and thereby allows deeper penetration of the fingers. Gently push your fingers into the restricted area to serve as an axis for manipulation. With your other arm, mobilize the patient posterosuperiorly, extending the spine in order to lengthen the fibers of the median umbilical ligament as much as possible *(Illustration 2-33)*. The technique should never be painful. Alternatively, the patient can lean back against you, while you also lean backward (for extension of the spine) and use both hands to pull upon the fibers of the median umbilical ligament.

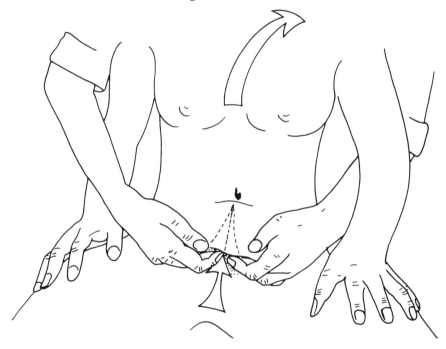

**Illustration 2-33**
Manipulation of Median Umbilical Ligament: Seated Position

Add a rotational component to treat the medial umbilical ligaments; this will enhance their degree of stretching. Do this before the backward bending. When the trunk is maximally rotated, the ligaments are stretched like cords. Repeat this technique gently and rhythmically about ten times to obtain a release.

SUPINE POSITION:  For a direct technique, bend the patient's legs and place your fingers over the area of restriction. If the restriction is halfway between the umbilicus and pubis, you can maintain it with one hand and stretch the surrounding tissues. You can also fix the subumbilical region and stretch the suprapubic region inferiorly, or fix the suprapubic region and stretch the subumbilical region superiorly. Lengthen the medial umbilical ligaments by stretching them in an oblique direction from bottom to top, right to left, etc. For a very effective combined technique, fix the area of restriction with one hand and rotate the bent legs with the other. Your two hands work in harmony as the legs are rotated left and right *(Illustration 2-34)*. Repeat this 4-5 times until your abdominal hand feels a release.

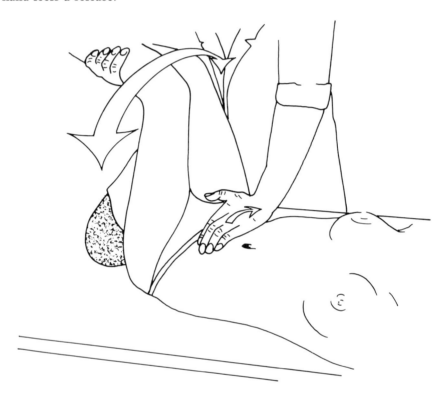

**Illustration 2-34**
Manipulation of Median Umbilical Ligament: Supine Position

KNEE / ELBOW POSITION:  This is an excellent position for manipulation of the median umbilical ligament. The patient rests on her forearms and you stand to one side. Maintain the restricted area with one hand; with the other, push on and rotate the sacrum *(Illustration 2-35)*. The median and medial umbilical ligaments will be strongly stretched, and you may feel microadhesions break up under your fingers. This technique should be painless, but do not repeat it more than 3-4 times.

MODIFIED TRENDELENBURG POSITION:  An advantage of this position is that it enables you to work easily with both hands. You can vary the slope using an adjustable table. For better results with a lateral area, have the patient place one foot upon the opposite thigh; this allows good access to the abdomen and upper suspensory structures of the bladder.

STANDING POSITION:  The patient stands and rests her forearms on the table. Stand behind her with both hands behind the symphysis, and pull upward to free fibrosed

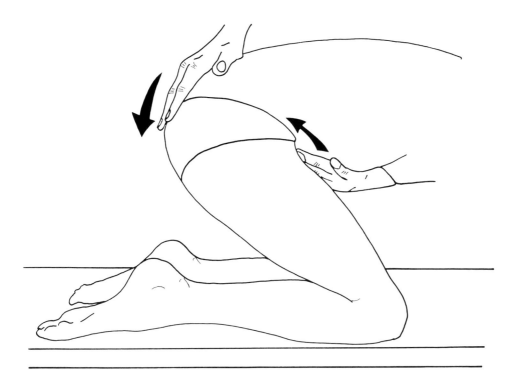

**Illustration 2-35**
Manipulation of Median Umbilical Ligament: Knee/Elbow Position

tissues. The patient should be bent forward slightly to relax the abdominal muscles. You may have to repeat this technique twelve times or so before a release is felt.

## Pubovesical Ligaments and Vesical Body

SUPINE POSITION: To relax the abdominal muscles, you can encourage hip flexion by placing a cushion under the patient's feet (legs bent), holding her knees near the abdomen with one hand, or (particularly for the lateral regions) placing one of her feet on the opposite thigh. Next, rhythmically push your fingers as far as possible under the pubis until you feel a release of the retracted fibers (Illustration 2-36).

The more medial your fingers are, the harder it will be to push them down. The pubovesical ligaments are tightest medially, as are the attachments of the abdominal muscles, linea alba, external inguinal canal, etc. To avoid having to "fight" these attachments, approach this region via the lateral edge of the rectus abdominis. If the patient has a diastasis of the linea alba, take advantage of it. Once your fingers are in place, rotate them back and forth until they are well under the pubis. The posterior side of the pubis is in contact with the prevesical space and bladder. In this region are found the insertions of the pubovesical ligaments and tendinous supports of the bladder wall muscles, as well as the pudendal venous plexus. If there is a fibrosis in the retropubic region, the bladder remains pressed against the pubis and cannot undergo its posteroinferior motion

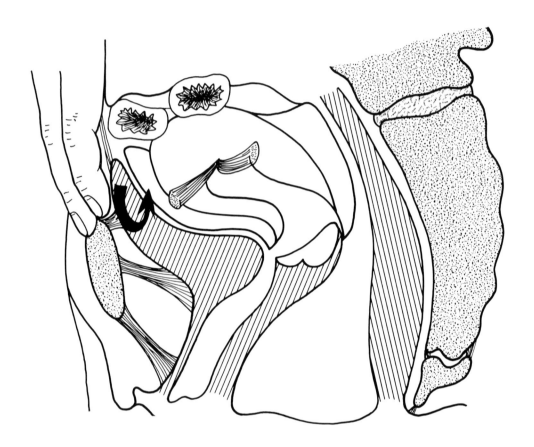

**Illustration 2-36**
Manipulation of Pubovesical Ligaments: Supine Position

in the sagittal plane. It is very important to release any excess tension in this area. Restrictions are often unilateral. Compare the two sides of the body to identify the restriction.

Although there is no definitive proof, we believe that freeing restricted structures in this region has a beneficial effect on the pudendal venous plexus. We have obtained immediate results in some cases of stress incontinence which are difficult to explain simply by restoration of sagittal motion. The more the patient's hips are flexed, the more deeply your fingers will be able to penetrate. Rotate and sidebend the knees; this will enhance the degree of stretching.

KNEE / ELBOW POSITION: In this position, the abdominal muscles are relaxed, and the small intestine and omentum are disengaged from the subpubic region. Place your fingers well under the pubis, stretch the fibrosed structures, and utilize hip flexion.

MODIFIED TRENDELENBURG POSITION: Flex the patient's hips and approach the subpubic region along both lateral edges of the rectus abdominis. Form your fingers into a spoon shape as if to surround the bladder. Pull on the bladder area while moving your leg to increase the degree of stretching *(Illustration 2-37)*. This technique permits general bladder mobilization and is effective for lateral parts of the bladder.

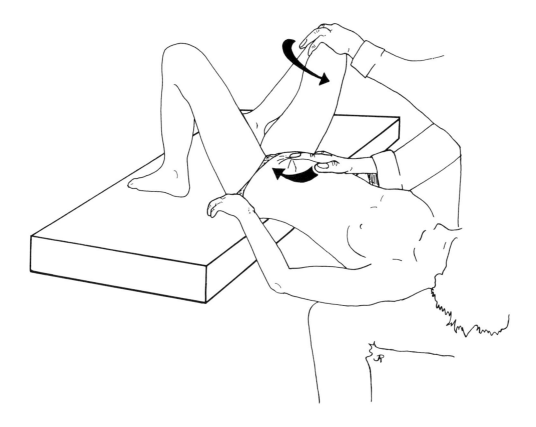

**Illustration 2-37**
Manipulation of Pubovesical Ligaments: Modified Trendelenburg Position

SEATED POSITION: Position your fingers along the iliopubic rami. Press them inward at first to get behind the pubis; then, gradually push them downward and inward *(Illustration 2-38)*. Because the abdominal muscles are relaxed and the spine flexed, you should be able to go deeply behind the pubis. For a unilateral iliopubic restriction, cross the legs such that the knee of the restricted side is on top. This technique is not advisable for patients with ptosed bladders because it tends to provoke incontinence.

## Subpubic Ligament

This is a fascial thickening which reinforces the pubic ligament found on the anterior ischiopubic ramus. To treat this ligament and stimulate vesical and perivesical reflexes, press upon the inferior part of the pubis and then upward to the anterior part, 3-4 times.

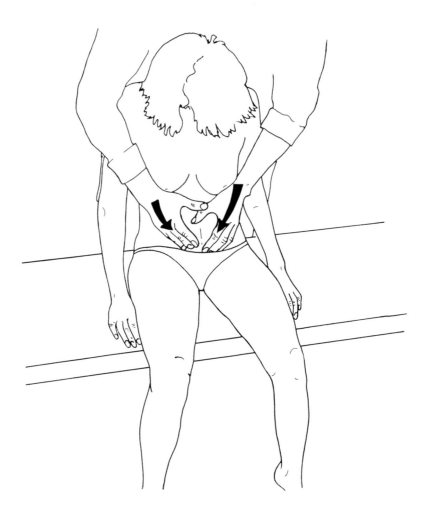

**Illustration 2-38**
Manipulation of Pubovesical Ligaments: Seated Position

### Anterior Perineum

This part of the perineum interacts closely with the bladder. To defibrose the preischial part of the perineal body, place your fingers on either side of the anterior vulva and labia majora (keeping them closed), then push slightly posteroinferolaterally *(Illustration 2-39)*. This will stretch the superficial perineal aponeurosis, urogenital diaphragm, bulbocavernosus, ischiocavernosus, and superficial transverse perineal muscles. This region always needs work after large episiotomies. This technique directly affects upon the pudendal nerves via the bulbospongiosus muscle and superficial perineum, situated between the labia minora and majora.

### Pubo-urethral Ligaments

Although a vaginal approach is more effective, you can also treat the inferior fibers of the pubo-urethral ligaments using an external approach. Keeping the anterior vulva

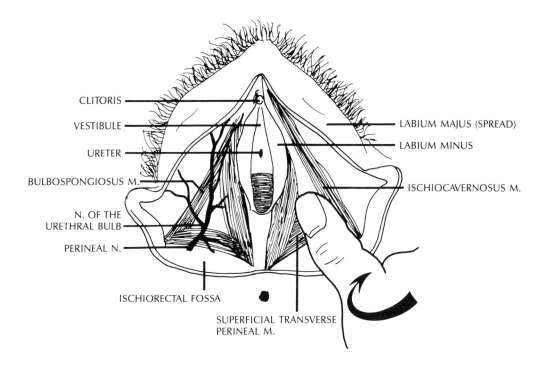

CLITORIS

VESTIBULE

URETER

BULBOSPONGIOSUS M.

N. OF THE
URETHRAL BULB

PERINEAL N.

LABIUM MAJUS (SPREAD)

LABIUM MINUS

ISCHIOCAVERNOSUS M.

ISCHIORECTAL FOSSA

SUPERFICIAL TRANSVERSE
PERINEAL M.

**Illustration 2-39**
Manipulation of Anterior Perineum

and labia majora closed, push your fingers under the pubis so that they press against the posterior side. Be careful to avoid the clitoral hood. Stretch the anterior pubo-urethral ligament attachments by drawing the fibers against the pubis.

## Obturator Foramen

Fluoroscopy has revealed the effectiveness of manipulation of the obturator foramen during bladder treatment. Pressure on the obturator can elevate a ptosed bladder by 2cm. No such effect was observed with pressure slightly lower down, on the adductor magnus. There are three possible explanations for this phenomenon:

- pressure on the obturator membrane increases perivesical cavitary pressure, which pushes the bladder upward;
- pressure on the obturator membrane is mechanically relayed to the bladder via the internal and external obturators and levator ani, and causes the bladder to contract;
- there is a nervous reflex system beginning with afferent nerve endings around the obturator and ending with efferent nerves to the suspensory structures of the bladder.

SUPINE POSITION:  The patient's hips are flexed, and the leg on the treated side is in abduction and slighlty externally rotated. Place your hand under the anterior adductors, thumb under pectineus and adductor magnus, index finger on gracilis. As you adduct and internally rotate the leg, slide your fingers around the adductors until your thumb is in contact with the external obturator, obturator membrane, and internal obturator. First you pronate, and, at the end, supinate your thumb. Wiggle your thumb slightly so that it is as close as possible to the obturator foramen, and stretch the tissues. Test both foramina and compare them. To increase penetration of the thumb, adduct and internally rotate the hip joint to release the pectineus, adductor longus, and pubofemoral ligament. Combine flexion, extension, abduction, and adduction movements to stretch and release the region; move your thumb further toward the head with each release *(Illustration 2-40)*. Ask the patient to isometrically contract her adductors so that you can feel their superior attachments and position your fingers optimally.

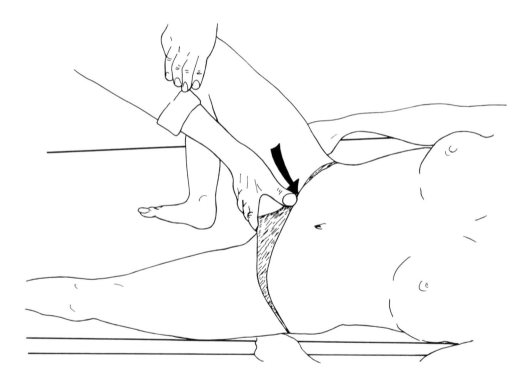

**Illustration 2-40**
Manipulation of Obturator Foramen

Once you have some competence in this difficult technique, you can utilize diaphragmatic respiration in your treatment. At the end of exhalation, if one obturator region is more tense than the other, the manipulation was not completely successful. To enhance the effectiveness of the treatment, at the end, put one thumb in each obturator foramen and balance the membranous tension between them. When checking both foramina, have both hips internally rotated and put your shoulders between the patient's knees.

It can be very useful to combine manipulation of the obturator foramen with that of the median and medial umbilical ligaments. One way of doing this is to push via the obturator foramen and pull gently on the median umbilical ligament until you feel the forces focused on the restricted area of the bladder. This can then be released, either by repeating the procedure gently and rhythmically, or by unwinding it.

STANDING POSITION: With severe bladder ptoses, it is better to test the obturator foramen with the patient standing so that gravity has its normal effect. The patient stands with her legs slightly apart and you follow the cord of the adductors as described above. When your thumb is correctly positioned, have the patient breathe out or cough slightly. A restricted area will only allow slight depression. This technique requires great confidence on the part of the patient.

STIMULATION OF OBTURATOR NERVE: For manipulation of the anterior perineum, your hand moves from the pubic symphysis toward the coccyx. The obturator nerve is located about three fingers' width from the symphysis down the iliopubic ramus *(Illustration 2-41)*. Stimulation of this nerve increases tonicity of the entire pelvic area, which can be very helpful in cases of hypotonia of the bladder and sphincters. Pluck the nerve gently as if it were a thin guitar string. In cases of knee pain or bladder hypertonia, simply inhibit the nerve.

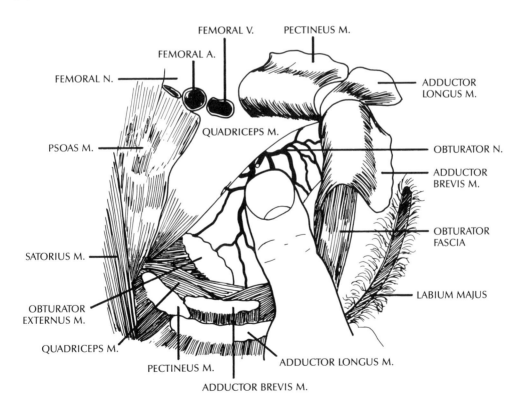

**Illustration 2-41**
Stimulation of Obturator Nerve

Some reflex knee pains related to problems of the uterus or bladder involve this nerve. An abnormal parietal stimulation directly stimulates a branch of the nerve leading to the adductor longus, from which an anterior branch runs to the synovial membrane of the knee. The posterior branch of the obturator nerve supplies the external obturator and adductor magnus. Abnormal stimulation of this branch often provokes adduction and external rotation of the leg. The obturator nerve can be stimulated by pressing on it gently 5-6 times. We have found this helpful in cases of ptosis.

GRYNFELT'S SPACE: This is bounded by the posterior and inferior serratus muscle, lateral edge of the paraspinal muscles, internal oblique, and rib 12. Grynfelt's space is an effective reflexogenic zone also used for restrictions of the kidneys. Simple digital compression here may be sufficient to restore mobility to a kidney. The left Grynfelt's space corresponds to the stomach, small intestine, or (less frequently) left kidney; the right is more specific to the kidneys and bladder. We presume that stimulation here acts via the nerves of the lumbar plexus. The subperitoneal tissues are in direct nervous communication with perimuscular tissues of the bladder. Stimulation should be repeated 3-4 times. This technique is useful in cases where the bladder has been fixed for a long time.

## COMBINED EXTERNAL AND VAGINAL TECHNIQUES

This is a typical bimanual approach using one abdominal hand and two intravaginal fingers. Move your abdominal hand toward the intravaginal fingers so that the tissues slide upon each other and restrictions and adhesions become obvious (Illustration 2-42). Once these are discovered, stretch the tissues from top to bottom, left to right, right to left, and circularly.

Check each plane with care, since a restriction may go unnoticed even when the fingers are right on it. The abdominal fingers move posteroinferiorly between the pubis and uterine fundus (if the position of the uterus allows this) and then the pubic symphysis. Be careful not to irritate the uterine tubes or ovaries. If you feel an ovary, immediately relax your pressure. Inappropriate pressure on an ovary usually produces pain and generalized spasms that make further treatment impossible. Remember, this is the same as having one's testicle squeezed.

One early success using bimanual technique encouraged us to pursue our work with urogenital manipulation. The patient had undergone surgery for a prolapsed bladder four times without success. She had suffered incontinence and a series of urinary tract infections for over four years. After one bimanual treatment for bladder unfolding, the infections ceased and continence improved. Unfortunately, most of our results are not this spectacular. A surprising aspect of this case was that there was no difference between cystographies done before and after treatment. Only the improvement in the patient's health and the disappearance of infection demonstrated the effectiveness of the treatment. We think that the bladder was folded posteriorly because we had an impression of unfolding during manipulation. These folds often harbor bacteria or other pathogens. With some unfolding techniques, one hears a crackling noise as the tissues are released.

For bladder neck prolapse, wedge your intravaginal finger in the anterior vaginal pouch (if it exists) or on the upper part of the anterior vaginal wall. The abdominal fingers, placed posterior to the symphysis, move toward the intravaginal fingers; both hands

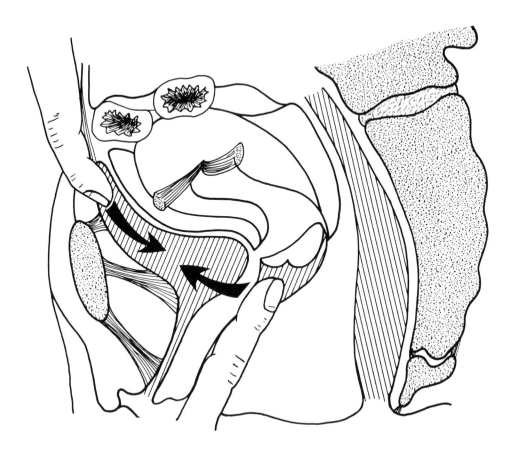

**Illustration 2-42**
Manipulation of Bladder: Bimanual Approach

then move superiorly and slightly posteriorly 4-5 times *(Illustration 2-43)*.

## VAGINAL TECHNIQUES

One can use these techniques to manipulate the trigonal/neck and pubo-urethral regions utilizing the anterior vaginal wall, vesicovaginal septum, vesicovaginal fascia, posterior urethral walls, and trigonal region as intermediaries.

### Bladder Neck Region

Restrictions here are easily found by pressing the vaginal septum toward the symphysis. We have observed that this region often presents restrictions in cases of postpartum dyspareunia or incontinence. Posterior projection or inflammation of the bladder neck can be treated by restoring normal mobility via manipulation of the anchoring tissues. Push the neck region anterolaterally and let it return. Repeat this rhythmically about 10 times. Then, place the fingers immediately below the neck to pull it anteriorly

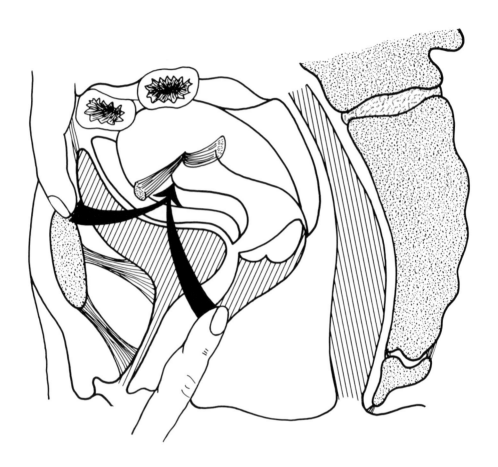

**Illustration 2-43**
Manipulation of Bladder Neck Prolapse

*(Illustration 2-44)*. The effectiveness of this technique may be due to direct effects on the tissues and/or stimulation of sympathetic nerves.

With severe restrictions of this region, first ask the patient to push her bladder down in order to enhance and clarify your perception. Next, ask her to hold her bladder in, and push the trigonal/neck region anterosuperiorly.

## Urethral Region

Like all tubes, the urethra must maintain a degree of elasticity to be functional. Also, the periurethral tissues transmit abdominal/pelvic pressures to baroreceptors and tonoreceptors around the urethra. For manipulation, place your fingers directly under the trigonal region and draw the uterus toward the body of the bladder while keeping the bladder tight against the pubis *(Illustration 2-45)*. This allows release of pubo-urethral and urethrovaginal adhesions, and the urethral lengthening has a reinforcing effect on tonus of the lumen. We often use a hand on the abdomen to give the treatment a more systemic effect. While performing this technique, always verify the position of the cervix, its tonicity, and the state of the parametrium.

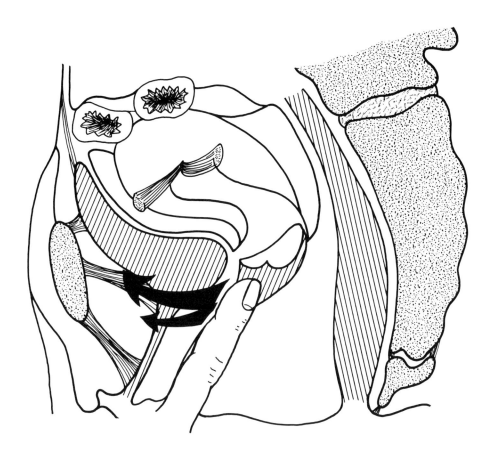

**Illustration 2-44**
Bladder Neck Manipulation

## INDIRECT TECHNIQUES

These techniques utilize the muscles which link the pelvis to the legs. Fluoroscopy has shown us that stretching techniques for leg muscles affect bladder position and tonicity. The bladder is able to contract through action of various pelvitrochanteric muscles (chiefly external rotators and abductors): internal obturator, external obturator, pyramidal, gemellus, and quadratus femoris. These muscles have direct or indirect insertions on the obturator membrane via the internal obturator tendon, the ischium, or the sciatic spine.

### Stretching and Toning the Pelvitrochanteric Muscles

In order to stretch the contiguous bladder/obturator regions, place the patient in supine position, the leg on the treated side above the other leg and drawn passively into internal rotation and adduction *(Illustration 2-46)*. This technique is useful for hypotonic bladders which have decreased mobility or are fixed (these are a common source of

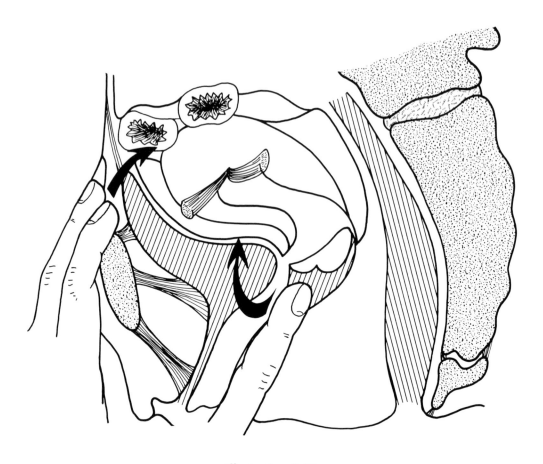

**Illustration 2-45**
Urethral Manipulation

infections and adhesions). Repeat this technique about 15 times, bilaterally. We believe that stretching the adductors has a slight effect upon the bladder, but have not confirmed this by fluoroscopy.

Toning of the pelvitrochanteric muscles is done by isometric contraction. The patient should perform, against opposition, alternating adductions of the two legs, progressively increasing the time of contraction. We observed under fluoroscopy that static contractions were more effective than dynamic movements. These exercises should be repeated 2-3 times a day, in the supine or standing position.

## Toning the Perineum

We have found perineal exercises helpful when associated with other techniques described here. During a perineal contraction, the urogenital organs move upward 2-3cm. Various manuals have described techniques for perineal tonification, mostly based on contractions of the gluteal, pelvitrochanteric, and abdominal muscles. In the technique we have found most helpful, the patient is supine, pelvis tilted backward and legs slightly

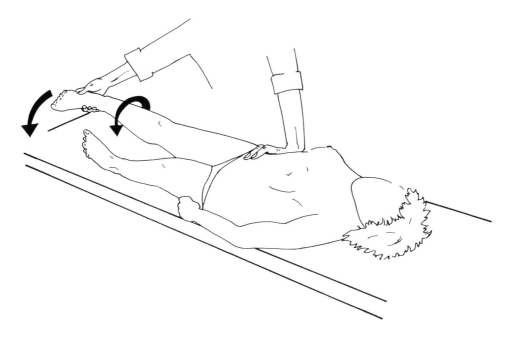

**Illustration 2-46**
Stretching the Pelvitrochanteric Muscles

apart. She makes a conscious urine-retention effort while pressing the external edges of her feet against the ground and contracting the gluteal muscles, as if pushing the pubis upward. A work-out of the perineum should always be combined with leg exercises, e.g., isometric contraction of the adductors. While contracting the perineum, the patient clasps a book tightly between the knees. This exercise can be repeated about 30 times, twice a day.

## Toning the Sphincters

This technique stimulates the urethral sphincters and increases the patient's awareness of them. Ask the patient to consciously and repeatedly interrupt urination. This will sensitize local and central nervous control and reinforce the occlusive role of the sphincter fibers. In addition, ask her to perform a pushing effort (as if to initiate urination) and then prevent it at the last second. This stimulates the detrusor and immediately releases it by contraction of the external sphincter.

## RECTAL TECHNIQUES AND THE COCCYX

The sacrococcygeal joint requires careful evaluation. It is most commonly fixed anteriorly (from falls on the buttocks), but can also be restricted posteriorly (following childbirth) or superiorly (from direct impact). Anterior restrictions, by relaxing the entire posterior uterovesical attachment system, disrupt mechanical occlusion of the bladder. Relaxation of the posterior vesicovaginal retinaculum produces type P incontinence, with collapse of the bladder.

Internal manipulation of the coccyx is most effectively performed via the rectum. You will need a well-lubricated glove. Although the knee/elbow position is commonly used, we prefer the prone position with legs slightly apart. This requires greater precision on your part but is less embarrassing for the patient. Gently press your index finger (palmar surface up) into the anus; if resistance is too strong, wait a moment but do not remove the finger. Pull gently on the anal sphincter to make it contract; then, at the moment when it relaxes, delicately move the finger in. Once past the sphincter, your job is easier. Push the finger first from back to front in order to move it upward, and then slightly from front to back. When the finger is correctly positioned, the sacrococcygeal joint is on the palmar surface (*Illustration 2-47*).

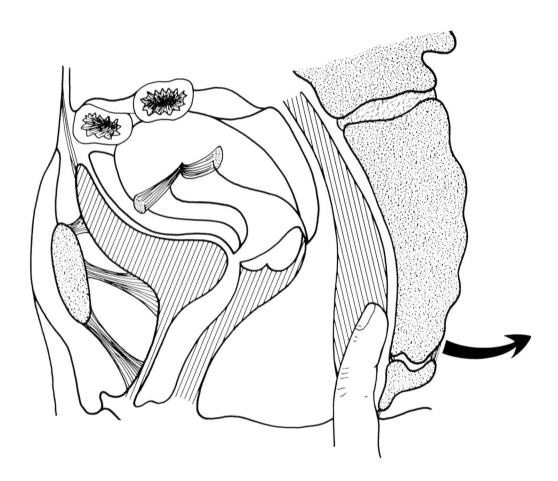

**Illustration 2-47**
Sacrococcygeal Manipulation: Rectal Route

While in this position, take a moment to check for hemorrhoids and to test the cervix, which is located perpendicular to the sacrococcygeal line when the finger is bent. If the cervix is retroflexed (although the prone position should anteflex it), you will immediately feel it against the anterior rectal septum. Push it anteriorly and feel it return. This is a good test of its mobility.

## Anteroposterior Manipulation

Stretch the coccygeal ligaments between the intrarectal finger and the thumb pressing upon the same spot externally. This is aided by pressing upon the sacrum with the other hand.

- If the anterior ligaments are fixed, stretch the coccyx posteriorly using the index finger.
- If the posterior ligaments are fixed, stretch the coccyx anteriorly using the thumb and thenar eminence.

Let the coccyx return to where it was and start anew with each movement. Do not try to "put something back in place," but rather release the fibrosed zones. As these tissues release, you may hear a characteristic crackling sound.

## Precautions

Intrarectal manipulation often produces a strong urge to defecate. Let the patient know beforehand that this is normal and not a cause for concern. To be on the safe side, have her use the toilet just before treatment. When withdrawing the finger, move very slowly and ask the patient to contract the anal sphincter and gluteal muscles as the finger comes out. A relaxed and respectful attitude on your part will make the patient more relaxed and thereby increase the efficacy of your treatment.

## External General Manipulation

Sometimes it is necessary to manipulate the coccyx externally. This type of work is generally less precise than that done via the rectum. It is still useful and worth knowing. One useful general technique for the coccyx is done with the patient prone. Your hypothenar eminence is placed as close to the coccyx as possible. Push cephalad until you see the head move. When you feel the maximum tension, release suddenly. Respiratory assistance may be used.

Another technique is done with the patient seated. Place your index or middle finger against the coccyx with your forearm along the spine. Your other hand positions the body while slightly compressing the cranial vault so that the weight of the body is precisely focused on the area of sacrococcygeal restriction. Pull the coccyx and sacrum very gently cephalad and unwind. There are many other ways to treat the coccyx.

## Lateral Manipulation

The coccyx occasionally becomes fixed in sidebending position. These cases do not involve true displacement (as in anterior or posterior restrictions), but rather a lack of proper distensibility of the sacrospinous or sacrotuberous ligaments, or various muscles and fasciae associated with the lateral sacrococcygeal joint. Fibrosis of a single coccygeus muscle is a good example. With lateral restrictions, you can release the coccyx by various means, via either the ischium or coccyx.

Place the patient in the lateral decubitus position (side of the restriction towards the table) with the upper leg bent in the classic "lumbar roll" position. Take up a pressure point with your forearm upon the ischium, and adjust it superiorly and slightly anteriorly to work on the sacrotuberous ligament. The same technique is usually then done on the opposite side to be sure that the forces are equilibrated.

The patient is in prone position with a small cushion under the pelvis to protect the anterosuperior iliac spines. Cross your hands and take up double ischiatic pressure points with your palms pressing on the tuberosities. The manipulation is performed by separating your hands on either side of the coccyx. Alternatively, with the patient in the same position, stand behind the patient with your arm straight and your palm on the sacrococcygeal joint and your other hand stabilizing the ilium in question. Adjust the sacrococcygeal junction anteriorly and slightly superiorly, with a rotational component, as if trying to move the sacrum away from the ischia.

## Stretching

With any significant coccygeal restriction, ask the patient to perform stretching movements in the seated position, bringing the knees alternately toward the opposite shoulder. In the seated position, the lateral coccygeal structures are "prestretched." The flexion and adduction movements of the hip increase ischiatic separation and lengthen the fibers of the coccygeus.

## RECTOVAGINAL TECHNIQUE

This seldom-used technique is useful for adhesions and fibroses of the rectouterine pouch which fix the neck of the posterior vagina posteriorly and inferiorly. This tilts the uterovesical axis posteriorly, placing the bladder in a permanent pushing position. After placing fingers of your two hands in the vagina and rectum, mobilize the perineal body by sliding it from one finger to another, and then stretch the rectovaginal septum inferiorly, in the direction of the restriction. After 4-5 repetitions, push the septum superiorly while pressing upon the cervix, and repeat. This technique should only be used in cases of uterine retroflexion. If the rectovaginal septum seems to have no restrictions, leave it alone.

## DIAPHRAGMATIC EXHALATION TECHNIQUE

In the case of a severely fixed bladder, a sudden and intense exhalation movement of the diaphragm can bring the abdominal/pelvic attachment system into play. Pelvic organs are then drawn upward by diaphragmatic attraction, even more so because forced exhalation diminishes cavitary pressures.

Put the patient in supine position, hips and knees flexed. Stand at her head with a hand on each side of the manubrium. Ask her to breathe in and out deeply, and accompany the movement of the thoracic cage with both hands. Compress the thorax at the end of exhalation, and release it suddenly at the beginning of inhalation. This technique creates a significant subdiaphragmatic suction which mobilizes the abdominal and pelvic organs and their attachments. For bladder problems, we follow this up with a similar technique. Place one hand on the body of the sternum pointing inferiorly, and the other just above the pubic symphysis pointing superiorly. As the patient exhales, the two hands move posteriorly and toward each other, following the movement of the patient's body. The hands resist the movements of inhalation. After two or three cycles, release the pressure just at the beginning of inhalation. Because of reciprocal tension and turgor effect, the pressure exerted in this technique causes a fixed bladder to vibrate against its attachments. The two techniques described above have a synergistic effect when applied alternately, and prepare the tissues for more specific manipulations.

## INDUCTION

With listening, the hand is automatically drawn toward restricted zones. A restriction functions as a new, abnormal axis of movement. Normally, the motility of the bladder is an anteroposterior swing with superior sliding. As you feel your hand go in the direction of the restriction, slightly accentuate what you feel. As it swings back, just let it go. Repeat this many times and you will gradually feel the movement increase and rediscover its normal motility *(Illustration 2-48)*. This technique, called induction, is finished when your hand is no longer attracted to the area that was restricted.

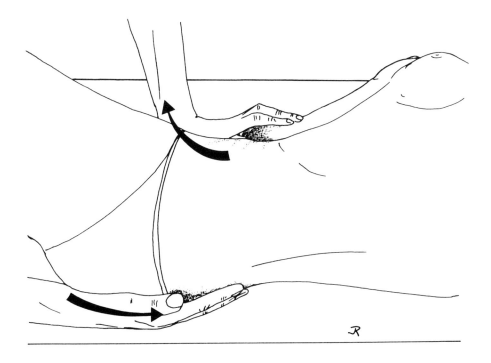

**Illustration 2-48**
Induction of Bladder

If you cannot feel the motion, recreate it several times as if you were cranking a car engine in an effort to restart it. Do this rhythmically, with a frequency around seven cycles per minute. With practice, you will be able to use motility or local listening for both diagnosis and precise treatment, forgetting traditional conceptions of ideal movement. Motility can thus be integrated into a general framework of global body motions. Let your fingers be your guide. After induction, recheck motility carefully. Our usual treatment strategy begins with listening, continues with mobility, and finishes with induction.

# Associated Restrictions

## VERTEBRAL COLUMN AND SKULL

The coccyx, due to its location, has close relationships with the bladder (as described above) and other pelvic organs. However, the entire vertebral column should be evaluated before testing and treatment of the bladder. Vertebral restrictions most commonly associated with bladder problems are those of T7, T11, L1, L2, and the sacrococcygeal joint—but do not ignore other segments! Osteopathy began with vertebral manipulation, and we should never neglect this regardless of which part of the body we are treating.

Cranial restrictions associated with problems of the vesical body and its superolateral attachments are rare; such problems are usually based on local mechanics. Such cranial restrictions as are encountered in such cases are typically frontal because of a "chain" of anterior membranous tension. On the other hand, if bladder problems are of the trigonal/neck area, posterior, or paracoccygeal, we frequently find restrictions of the posterior skull—occiput, occipitomastoid sutures, foramen magnum, and hypophyseal area of the sphenoid. You can feel the tension all along the posterior vertebral axis, notably when the sacrum is fixed in extension.

## LEGS

We often take the legs and feet for granted. However, restrictions here can be extremely pathogenic. Neglecting them can render any treatment, however skilled, unsuccessful.

Restrictions of the legs and feet are usually explained by the chain of fasciae, and the relentless force of gravity. Proximal and distal restrictions of the fibula are common. The bladder and its attachments depend upon the internal obturator and its aponeurosis. They share many fibers with the sacrospinous and sacrotuberous, which in turn exchange fibers with the biceps femoris. The latter inserts on the head of the fibula—one explanation for the lesional chain between the fibula and bladder. More rarely, bladder problems may be associated with restrictions of the distal tibiofibular joint, navicular bone, or the fifth metatarsal. In some cases, we have mobilized bladders (as verified by fluoroscopy) simply by pressing on the navicular, whereas the same pressure exerted on nearby sites provoked no movement at all. Always test both legs, even for a unilateral bladder restriction.

As the legs are so intimately related to the bladder, we strongly recommend that the appropriate leg muscles be stretched after treating the bladder. For example, the stretching of the internal obturator muscle ( see *Illustration 2-21* above) is usually done after bladder treatments. If the treatment was successful, the patient will feel no discomfort.

## REFLEXOGENIC ZONES

We have obtained good results with bladder problems by working with certain reflexogenic zones. The explanation may lie in their innervation, in muscle/fascial chains, or some unknown mechanism. There are many phenomena of the human body which we still do not understand. Work on these zones by digital massage of the ligaments and overlying skin, or by induction:

- lacunar ligament (part of the aponeurosis of the external oblique which forms the medial boundary of the femoral ring)
- Cooper's ligament (a fold of the transversalis fascia attached to the iliopectineal eminence and pubic spine)
- inguinal ligament
- sciatic spine
- lumbar triangle.

## *Results and Advice*

Bladder manipulations have clearly beneficial effects on stress incontinence. We have used and evaluated the techniques described here extensively, on hundreds of patients. Effects on incontinence are easily documented. The patient does or does not retain urine successfully. In approximately 70% of the cases we have treated, there was 50% or better improvement in continence; in half of these the problem was essentially resolved. Imagine the joy of a patient who sees even a 50% improvement in continence. Her everyday life changes profoundly. She can laugh, cough, get up from a chair, play sports, without fear.

We have also had good results with cystitis, cystalgia, and recurrent infections. However, our results in these cases are more difficult to quantify in terms of intensity and duration. The hormonal dependence of the trigonal/neck region is a confounding factor. We have observed that this region is more sensitive and unstable during ovulation and menstruation. Your chances of success will increase if you treat your patients during the week following the menstrual period. An estrogen/progesterone imbalance adversely affects proper functioning of this region. As osteopaths we can work with structural attachments and mobility of organs, but what can we do about the effects of menopause on hypothalamic-pituitary hormone secretion? We are similarly powerless to deal with a patient's social or psychological situation. For example, our treatments are less likely to be effective for a patient trapped in an abusive relationship, going through a divorce, etc.

The advice you give can enhance and lengthen the positive results of your manipulations. Advise your patient to:

- empty her bladder and rectum before the treatment;
- practice the modified Trendelenburg position at home, e.g., pelvis resting on a chair, legs on the chair back, shoulders on the floor;
- assure ample diaphragmatic movement during Trendelenburg exercises, and pull the superior bladder attachments by drawing the fingers from pubis to umbilicus during exhalation;
- contract the perineum by pushing the pubis forward while pushing the lateral edges of the feet against some resistance;
- tonify the external sphincter by deliberately and repeatedly interrupting urination;
- exercise the levators, e.g., by contraction of the vagina.

Pelvic pressures induced by coughing are enormous. Advise the patient that if she feels the need to cough or sneeze, she should lean on a chair or table, or stand with knees flexed and hands pressed against the thighs. These positions, well-known to sufferers of lower back pain, allow much of the pressure on the perineum to be transferred to the arms and legs. For patients with incontinence, contraction of the sphincters and perineal orifices can be reinforced by sitting with the legs crossed.

You may feel uncomfortable at first trying to give this sort of advice, or think that the patient will not follow it. Don't worry. The personal and interpersonal problems posed by incontinence are considerable, and when the patient sees the positive results from following your advice, that will be all the reinforcement that is needed.

# Chapter Three:
## The Uterus and Vagina

# Table of Contents

# The Uterus and Vagina

M any events and forces affect the uterus and its attachments, some related to its primary function, others not. They include pregnancy, childbirth, large episiotomies, suction, forceps, sedentary professions, primary or secondary hormonal imbalances, traumas, surgery, multiple infections, and genetic susceptibility to dysplasia.

Functioning of the uterus and vagina is closely interrelated with that of the bladder. In chapter 2 we discussed the social implications of bladder problems, and the value of osteopathic treatment. Avoiding surgery is equally important, and many problems of the uterus are amenable to our treatment. All too often women who suffer from a pelvic disorder see themselves condemned to the conventional regimen of painkillers and anti-inflammatory drugs until the inevitable trip to the surgical suite.

Manipulation of the uterus and its attachments can take place via external or internal routes. Both require great palpatory sensitivity, gentleness, respect, and understanding on your part. Always explain to the patient what you are doing. Some practitioners who are uncomfortable with this area get into long winded explanations to delay doing the work. This is as bad as no explanation at all. It is important that both you and the patient are relaxed.

As always, we urge you to regard the human body as a functioning whole, and not imagine that you can treat one part of it in isolation. The uterus and its surroundings are affected by, and have effects on, many other regions of the body.

## Visceral Articulations

We assume that you are familiar with the basic anatomy of the uterus, and the names of its parts and associated structures. The wonderful discipline of anatomy is the keystone of our art. We will limit ourselves here to a very brief description of some of the relations between the uterus and its neighboring structures *(Illustration 3-1)*.

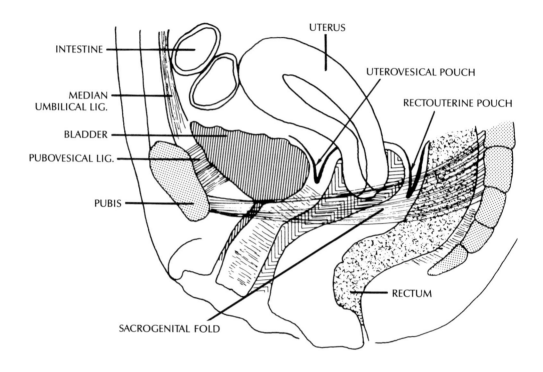

INTESTINE

MEDIAN
UMBILICAL LIG.

BLADDER

PUBOVESICAL LIG.

PUBIS

SACROGENITAL FOLD

UTERUS

UTEROVESICAL POUCH

RECTOUTERINE POUCH

RECTUM

**Illustration 3-1**
Relationships of the Uterus

The fundus (also known as the uterine base) is the rounded superior aspect of the uterus, covered by the peritoneum which clings tightly to it. This aspect of the uterus interacts with the small intestine and pelvic colon. The anteroinferior aspect of the part of the uterus below the fundus (called the body or corpus) is convex and covered by peritoneum as far as the isthmus, at which point the peritoneum reflects onto the superior bladder and forms the uterovesical pouch. The uterus as a whole is tilted forward (anteverted) so that it normally rests upon the bladder. The posterior uterus is covered by the peritoneum as far as the posterosuperior vagina, at which point the peritoneum reflects onto the anterior rectum and forms the rectouterine pouch (also known as Douglas' pouch).

The superolateral angles comprise the uterine "horns," where the uterine tubes lead out to the ovaries, and the round ligaments and ovarian ligaments attach. The lateral edges of the uterus are wide and rounded. The broad ligaments are peritoneal folds extending from the lateral uterus to the side walls of the pelvic cavity.

The cervix of the uterus, anteriorly, is related to the anterior vaginal wall and, through it, to the posterior bladder. Posteriorly, the cervix relates to the posterior vaginal wall, rectouterine pouch, and rectum. Laterally, it relates to the ureters, blood vessels, and pelvic subperitoneal space.

## SUSPENSION AND SUPPORT

There are numerous ligaments and other connective tissue structures suspending

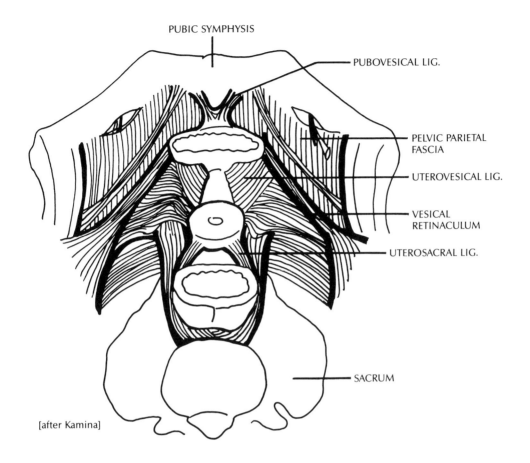

PUBIC SYMPHYSIS

PUBOVESICAL LIG.

PELVIC PARIETAL FASCIA

UTEROVESICAL LIG.

VESICAL RETINACULUM

UTEROSACRAL LIG.

SACRUM

[after Kamina]

**Illustration 3-2**
Uterus: Means of Connection

and supporting the uterus *(Illustration 3-2)*. As the astute reader will observe, these structures are closely interrelated with the attachments of the bladder.

The **peritoneum**, as in the case of the bladder, has a very minor role in suspending the uterus. However, peritoneal restrictions can seriously disrupt mobility of the uterus.

The **round ligaments** are thin fibrous cords that start from the uterine horns, run anterolaterally through the deep inguinal ring and inguinal canal, and finally break up into strands that merge into the labia majora. Near the uterus, this ligament contains many smooth muscle fibers; these progressively disappear farther away from the uterus. The round ligaments slightly antevert and stabilize the uterus. They have reflexogenic effects when manipulated.

The **broad ligaments** connect the uterus to the lateral walls of the internal pelvis. The superior portion is thin and mobile, while the inferior portion becomes progressively thicker. The posterior surface relates to the small intestine. Two levels can be considered. The superior level is reinforced by three arches at the level of the round and ovarian ligaments and uterine tube. The lower level is the parametrium. Here the broad ligament thickens and picks up fatty tissue intertwined with connective and muscular fibers. It interacts with the ureters and uterine blood vessels and, at a greater distance, with the anterolateral abdominal walls and iliolumbar region.

Many pelvic blood vessels have connective/muscular sheets anchoring them to nearby structures. Of particular interest are two structures primarily associated with the internal iliac artery, the **sacrogenital folds** (also known as the rectouterine folds). These run from the middle sacrum (S2, S3, S4) to the pubis, through the subperitoneal tissue space. Their anterior part goes from the isthmus to the anterior sacral foramen, and their posterior part has two reinforced sections called the uterosacral ligaments. The sacrogenital folds attach to the rectum, isthmus, superior vagina, and bladder, and contribute to the strong connection between these organs.

The **uterosacral ligaments** are the posterior reinforced sections of the sacrogenital folds which connect the uterus to the rectum and sacrum. They are attached at the level of the isthmus and prevent the cervix from moving toward the bladder and symphysis pubis. Their attachment is the "relative fixed point" of the uterus, about which anteversion and rotational movements take place.

The **pelvic floor** was discussed in chapter 2. It comprises many muscles (levator ani, internal obturators, pyramidalis, transverse perineal, bulbospongiosus, ischiocavernosus, sphincter ani), aponeuroses, and other connective tissues. It forms the inferior and lateral walls of the pelvic cavity, and plays an indispensable role in support and pressure distribution of the pelvic organs.

### Pelvic Stabilizing System

The uterus is held up, at the level of the isthmus, by a cross-shaped structure formed primarily by lateral parametrial anchorage to the pelvic floor, and by the sacrogenital folds *(Illustration 3-3)*. As this aspect of pelvic mechanics is concerned with stationary support instead of dynamic motion, it is also referred to as the "static" pelvis. We will describe the transverse and longitudinal elements of this structure separately.

TRANSVERSE ELEMENTS: These include the arches of the broad ligament:

- the interior arch orients the uterine body;
- the middle arch covers the uterine tubes and influences lateral stability of the uterus and mobility of the tubes and ovaries;
- the posterior arch is made up of the suspensory ovarian ligament which connects the ovary to the lateral pelvic wall, and the ovarian ligament which connects the ovary to the uterine horn.

The **parametrium** is composed of connective fibers inserting on the isthmus, the sides of the cervix, and the tendinous center of the broad ligament. The lateral uterosacral ligaments insert in the parametrium posteriorly, the pillar of the cervix inside, and the lateral pillar of the bladder anteriorly. The parametrium has some contractile capability and is crossed by numerous vessels.

The **precervical fascia** runs from the cervix to the uterovesical pouch and merges with the vesicovaginal fascia.

The **retrocervical fascia** is thinner, and connects to the uterosacral ligaments. Interlacing of this fascia forms a fold known as the torus uterinus.

LONGITUDINAL ELEMENTS: These are based on the sacrogenital folds and uterosacral ligaments and can be divided into several component parts.

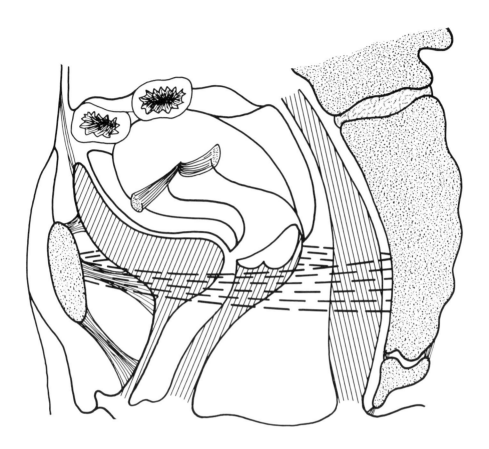

**Illustration 3-3**
Pelvic Stabilizing System

The **anterior part** includes the uterovesical ligaments or medial pillars of the bladder, which merge with the vesicovaginal fascia and pubovesical ligaments:

- the medial pillars of the bladder (uterovesical ligaments) are solid fibromuscular cords approximately 2.5cm thick;
- the lateral pillars of the bladder run from the tendinous center of the broad ligament to the vesical apex.

The **posterior part** consists of the uterosacral ligaments. These attach to the lateral wall of the rectouterine pouch. The uterosacral portion is relatively dense, thick, and muscular, while the vaginosacral portion is made of mostly collagenous fibers.

The **middle liaison system** links the superior and inferior levels, and consists of the vesicovaginal fascia and prerectal hemisheaths.

The **inferior part** consists of certain perineal muscles which function in support of the pelvis. The perineal body is an important element. Good support of the uterus depends on normal tonicity of these muscles.

## LOCALIZATION AND LANDMARKS

As the uterus is often treated in association with the bladder, we will also mention some landmarks for the bladder here. Locations of important structures are described here. Of course, there are variations among individuals.

- Pubovesical ligaments: attached to the upper and middle parts of the posterior side of the pubic symphysis.
- Pubo-urethral ligaments: attached to the bottom aspect of the symphysis.
- Bottom of the uterus: behind the symphysis, 2-3cm below the pelvic end of the rectus abdominis.
- Round ligaments: 10–12cm in length, diameter 3–6mm. Their anterior part is accessible across the inguinal canal, and the posterior part upon the lateral horns of the uterus (if these are accessible).
- Uterosacral ligaments: 6–7cm high. On the anterior aspect of S2-S4 and uterine isthmus.
- Broad ligaments: at the internal wall of the iliac fossa and around the cervix.
- Perineal body: a hard mass between the rectum and vagina. Felt by depressing the region between the anus and vulva.
- Vagina: the vagina and rectum are separated by the rectouterine pouch at the top 2cm of the vagina. The pelvic part (upper two-thirds) of the vagina relates to the parametrium. The rectovaginal septum is slack. The perineal part of the vagina, from top to bottom, relates to the internal fasciculi of the levators, pelvic aponeurosis, middle perineal aponeurosis, deep transverse perineal muscles, constrictor of the vulva, and vestibular bulb.
- Neck of the bladder: on a horizontal plane passing through the inferior part of the pubic symphysis and 2.5cm posteriorly. The bladder neck relates to the cervix.
- Cervix: on a horizontal plane passing through the sacrococcygeal joint. The supravaginal segment corresponds to the lower base of the bladder and the trigone. At rest, the cervix and bladder neck are at the same height. Even with great effort, they should not go past the transverse plane which goes through the coccyx.
- Uterine pouches: measuring 6mm anteriorly and 18mm posteriorly, the cervix being mostly covered at the back. The rectouterine pouch is 6–7cm from the anus, behind the cervix.
- Isthmus: in the center of the pelvic cavity. Its surface projection is at the height of the sciatic spine.
- Ureter and uterine artery: their crossover point is 15mm lateral to the bottom of the lateral vaginal pouch.
- Promontory: halfway between the umbilicus and symphysis.
- Umbilicus: at the bottom of L4, not at the level of L3 as is often taught.
- Aortic bifurcation: Between L4 and L5.

## SLIDING SURFACES

The uterus forms visceral articulations with the following nearby structures:

- superiorly with the peritoneum, small intestine, and colon, which can press upon it;

- anteriorly with the peritoneum and (via the uterovesical pouch) bladder. The small intestine can slide between the uterus and bladder when the bladder is empty.
- posteriorly with the peritoneum and (via the rectouterine pouch) rectum. With a retroverted uterus, there are more sliding surfaces here.
- laterally with the broad ligaments and subperitoneal pelvic tissue;
- inferiorly, the cervix/isthmus region articulates with the bladder neck/trigonal region, lower base of bladder, vagina, and perineal elements.

The uterus, despite its extraperitoneal position, is closely associated with the peritoneum and affected by disorders there. The peritoneal pouches (particularly rectouterine pouch) are typically affected by septic or mechanical irritations. Fibrosed pouches alter pelvic visceral mechanics and demand our attention. The superior part of the uterus requires harmonious tension of the peritoneum and numerous ligaments in the area; restrictions of these structures interfere with proper uterine movement. Loops of the small intestine which escape from the peritoneal cavity can press upon the uterus, make depressions in it, or even infiltrate between it and the other pelvic organs.

## Physical Examination and Diagnosis

The standard physical exam is described in all medical textbooks. There is no need to duplicate those discussions here. Take note of structural type, secondary sexual characteristics, anovulvular distance, and perineal scarring. Palpation permits evaluation of tonicity and elasticity of all pelvic tissues. Mobility and motility tests, and other specialized forms of palpation, will be described later. The pelvic exam lets you evaluate the mobility of the cervix and uterus, position of uterus, state of its adnexa, etc. The rectal exam lets you explore the parametrium, uterosacral ligaments, hemorrhoidal veins, and movements of the coccyx.

Many patients present with vague pains which are difficult to classify. The pelvic region is subject to numerous pathologies, some of which are quite serious. Anyone who works in this area should have at least one good, up-to-date textbook on gynecology and be very familiar with it. Do not risk missing a critical diagnosis. If you have the slightest doubt, refer the patient for appropriate testing or to a specialist.

### HISTORY

Whereas history-taking for stress incontinence is fairly simple, that for genital system problems requires great precision and thoroughness. Let the patient spontaneously describe her history and problems in her own words, with you providing direction or specific questions only when necessary. Do not get into a situation where you are asking a series of "yes or no" questions. History should cover age; profession; family history; date of first period; frequency of periods, duration of bleeding, infections; abortions; obstetrical, surgical, abdominal, back, urinary, intestinal problems; as well as any other significant disease or disorder which the patient has experienced.

## DYSMENORRHEA

Find out if dysmenorrhea is primary (appeared with the first period) or secondary (appeared later). Also determine the time of onset in relation to menstrual flow. *Premenstrual pain* can occur at the very beginning of menstrual flow (when it is intense and short-lasting), or it can begin the day before and not disappear until the flow is well established. This type of pain is usually related to fluid or venous congestion of the genital region from hormonal imbalances. It can also be due to intestinal spasms during the luteal phase. *Intermenstrual pain* appears in the middle of the period, becomes intense near the end, and disappears when blood flow stops. This type of pain can occur with endometriosis, problems of the uterine attachments, or ptosis. *Postmenstrual pain* does not start until near the end of the flow and may last one or a few days. It may also be secondary to endometriosis, but you must check for infections and lower back restrictions.

Find out if the pain is relieved by rest, if it disappears or increases at night, if it is discontinuous or continuous, if it is paroxysmal, of a weighty, pulling, radiating (to the lumbar, perineal, or obturator areas, or even frank sciatica) type, or accompanied by general symptoms such as vomiting, diarrhea, migraines, fainting, or emaciation. Take information about the flow (length, intensity, black or red blood, clots, smells, leucorrhea, pruritus), urinary problems, hemorrhoids, or anything else out of the ordinary.

## PELVIC PAINS

CYCLICAL PELVIC PAINS: Usually either manifestations of a central hormonal problem with local repercussions, or of a local problem. For example, the pain of a tumor can often be aggravated by premenstrual pelvic congestion.

NONCYCLICAL PELVIC PAINS OF EXTRAGENITAL ORIGIN: These include rheumatological or articular problems that project to the pelvis via secondary reflex stimulation. Pains of this type can also be secondary to urinary problems such as disturbance of bladder neck/trigonal mechanics, infections, stones, hydronephrosis, or renal tuberculosis. Cervical cancer can sometimes spread to the bladder. Pelvic pain caused by digestive system problems is sometimes difficult to distinguish from that due to genital problems. Examples are interposed rectum, rectal hemorrhage, tenesmus, violent colic, constipation, diarrhea, hemorrhoids, injury to the small intestine, adhesions, hernias, and enteritis.

NONCYCLICAL PELVIC PAINS OF GENITAL ORIGIN: You need to get specific information on depth and intensity of *dyspareunia* (pain related to intercourse). Superficial dyspareunia is localized just inside the vagina, most commonly as the sequela of an episiotomy. It is usually secondary to trauma of the middle perineal prevulval layer, rather than real tears. Another possible cause is excessively tight myorrhaphy of the levators for treatment of prolapse. Superficial vaginismus is sometimes seen in girls or young women. In menopausal women, this type of pain may indicate vulval atrophy of genital involution. Other more rare cases include herpes, eczema, and polyps in the orifice. Spasms of the levators may be a psychologically-based problem.

Dyspareunia can also result from changes in the vaginal tissues, due either to local problems (e.g., vaginitis from various organisms; vaginal involutive atrophy) or systemic problems (e.g., Sjögren syndrome).

Pain may also occur only during deep penetration. This can be due to a tear of the cervix combined with uterine retroversion, to what is known as the "Masters and

Allen syndrome," or to endometriosis affecting the broad or uterosacral ligaments. With the Masters and Allen syndrome, during clinical examination one finds: retroversion, a painful hypermobility provoked at the insertion points of the ligaments (often more intense on one side), and tearing of the posterior layer of the broad ligament with possible extension to the peritoneum and rectouterine pouch.

In our experience, deep dyspareunia usually has a mechanical origin, not a psychosomatic origin. You should try to get complete information in cases of dyspareunia, while still allowing the patient to feel relaxed. The better you understand the problem, the more precise and effective your treatment can be. It is also necessary to check for problems in the partner, such as Peyronie's disease.

The position in which pain occurs can help you determine which structures are involved.

- In the *prone position*: pain at the beginning of penetration can indicate a urethral or bladder neck/trigonal problem (e.g., ptosis, bladder inflammation), or significant genital prolapse. Pain at the end of penetration can indicate cervicitis, anteversion or anteflexion of the uterus, or anterior displacement of the cervix.
- In the *supine position*: pain at the beginning can indicate a prolapse; at the end, retroversion or retroflexion of the uterus, or adhesions of the parametrium.
- In the *lateral decubitus position*: pain at the end can indicate sidebending of the uterus with a tear of the broad ligament. In these cases, simply lying in the lateral decubitus position may be painful.

## INFECTIONS

There are many infectious agents that attack this area of the body. Infections can be acute or chronic, and involve any of the internal or external urogenital organs or openings. Be alert for the presence of sexually transmitted diseases. These can have serious consequences, including sterility. If you have any reason to suspect a sexually transmitted disease, send the patient for complete lab testing. Always check the abdomen carefully to see if it is hard with painful mobilization, which could be the sign of an infection affecting the peritoneum. Whenever in doubt, refer the patient to a specialist.

## MALIGNANT TUMORS

The genital system is a frequent site of tumor development, and you should always be on the lookout for signs such as unexplained masses, inter-menstrual bleeding, repeated discharge, night pains unrelated to the menstrual cycle, or any precisely located premenstrual pain. If you suspect a tumor, send the patient for a complete examination, including x-rays. Do not be deterred by imagined dangers of radiation exposure. It is worth the small risk of a few rads to save a life.

## UTERINE FIBROMA (LEIOMYOMA)

When there are significant uterine fibromas the uterine body feels like a fairly firm mass. This mass is mobile in every direction and is dull when percussed. Mobilization of the uterus primarily occurs at the level of the cervix. The sign is very clear-cut. Under your finger you can feel the cervix move depending on the push from the fibroma. Watch out for softening of the cervix or of the uterine body, which are signs of pregnancy. There is usually a feeling of small lumps in the uterus itself, the number and size differing from one patient to the next. A fibroma can be lumpy while at the same time keeping a firm consistency and the impression of movement with palpation and mobilization, in conjunction with the uterine body.

One interesting point is that pain and discomfort vary enormously. A patient with an enormous fibroma may be totally asymptomatic. Sometimes a small fibroma is harder to tolerate than a large one.

A fibroma is not a contraindication for internal manipulation as long as it is not aggressive. If internal techniques provoke bleeding, you obviously need to alter your approach.

## PAINFUL UTERINE RETROVERSION

Retroversion means rotation of the uterus in a posterior direction *(Illustration 3-4)*. Pelvic examination demonstrates the retroversion and ligamentous pain which is often

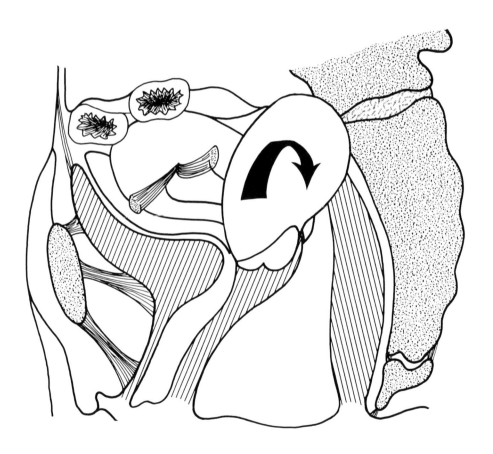

**Illustration 3-4**
Uterine Retroversion

unilateral, due to a tear of the posterior layer of the broad ligament. Major retroversion can cause a wide array of problems, as follows.

PAIN: This is often unilateral, and may occur in the pelvic, lumbar, or sacrococcygeal areas. The patient feels as if a foreign body or a weight is inside her. There may be a feeling of pressure in the rectal area. Pain is increased when standing up, walking, or fatigued. It is relieved by rest, particularly in the prone or knee/elbow position. The patient always tries to ease the pain by holding up her stomach.

DYSPAREUNIA: The pain is immediate and intense, and may be aggravated by deep penetration or orgasm.

DYSMENORRHEA: Pain associated with menstruation is relieved in the prone, knee/elbow, or modified Trendelenburg position. Changing position will either decrease or aggravate the pain.

CIRCULATORY PROBLEMS: The pelvis is congested, and the uterus is purplish-blue and edematous. There are often varicose veins of the legs. These are usually unilateral, perhaps reflecting a unilateral restriction of the uterus.

DIGESTIVE AND URINARY PROBLEMS: Common digestive symptoms are constipation and painful defecation. Common urinary problems are a sense of increased bladder weight, frequent urination, and dysuria.

ARTICULAR RESTRICTIONS: The sacrum is either strongly fixed anteriorly (no possibility of movement), fixed in anterior flexion, or, more rarely, in sidebending to the side opposite to the tear of the broad ligament.

## PAIN RELATED TO UTERINE STASIS

POSTERIOR DISPLACEMENT: This causes pelvic pain, low back pain, sciatica (rarely going farther than halfway down the thigh), rectal pain, and dyspareunia. A prolapse gives a characteristic stretching sensation.

ANTERIOR DISPLACEMENT: This causes mostly pelvic pain, bladder pain, heavy sensation in the bladder, and urinary problems.

COMPRESSION: This can be due to pregnancy, fibromas, cancer, or any invasion of the lower pelvis. Any of these can cause low back pain with a sensation of heaviness and abdominal discomfort. Pain sometimes radiates to the groin and thigh.

We have seen several cases of neuralgia involving the leg which could have led us to suspect a mechanical pathology of the hip joint, with painful limitation to articular movement. Good internal and lumbar manipulation (when there is a joint restriction), immediately improves the pain limits of the hip joint. This kind of treatment can give spectacular results!

# *Movement*

The healthy uterus is mobile, under the control of several passive and active factors.

## PASSIVE MOVEMENTS

### Respiratory Diaphragm

The strong, rhythmic contractions of the diaphragm mobilize all the abdominal and pelvic organs. Its effects diminish with distance, but nonetheless influence the uterus. Forced inhalation and exhalation can move the bottom of the uterus 2cm in a young woman. In the knee-chest position, the liver, intestinal mass and other sub-diaphragmatic elements press against the diaphragm, creating a relative negative pressure in the pelvis. Although the effect is difficult to quantify, some studies suggest that the "attractive" force of the diaphragm reduces the effective weight of the uterus by approximately 50%.

### Walking

Walking, getting into or out of a chair, and other everyday activities cause the uterus to passively follow the body's movements. This promotes the natural and healthy mobility of the uterus. Simple inactivity, even without a structural problem, can reduce mobility and thereby predispose parts of the uterus to inflammation or other disorders.

### Influence of Bladder and Rectum

When the bladder is full, all of its diameters (especially the vertical) increase. This pushes the uterine fundus superiorly and slightly posteriorly. If the uterus is, for example, retroverted and anteflexed, the pressure from a full bladder will be focused on the cervix, leading to tension in this area. If the tension is strong enough, the bladder may be passively depressed by the cervix.

When the rectum is full, the uterus is pushed forward. This commonly happens in women with persistent constipation affecting the lower colon. If the bladder and rectum are simultaneously full, their forces combine to lift up and verticalize the uterus. You should find out whether pain is eased when the bladder is full, or just before defecation.

Pushing (to empty the bladder or rectum) or retention movements have characteristic effects on the uterus and vagina:

- when pushing *(Illustration 3-5)*, the anchorage systems relax and the urethral and uterovaginal angles ("vaginal cap") disappear. The bladder base and cervix/isthmus region move slightly posteroinferiorly, pressing upon the superior half of the posterior vagina. The uterus and vagina press upon the rectum, and the rectouterine pouch is closed.
- when retaining, the anterior anchorage system contracts while the posterior anchorage system remains fixed. This causes the vaginal cap to increase and the pouches to open.

Pushing and retention movements are mostly passive and due to variations in abdominal or perineal pressure, and to the attachment system of the pelvis. Tonus of the abdominal wall, bladder, and uterus affect these movements.

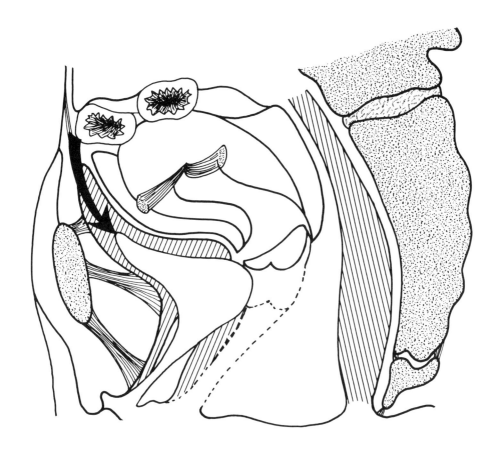

**Illustration 3-5**
Pushing Movements

# INTRINSIC OR ACTIVE MOVEMENTS

## Hormonal Rhythm

The position of the uterus changes in response to the menstrual cycle, events such as puberty and menopause, and general physical condition. In a young woman, a retroverted uterus changes position before and after each period.

Before ovulation, estrogen increases tonus of the myometrium and frequency of contractions, and interstitial fluid absorption increases, with a resulting increase in the weight of the uterus. In the luteal phase, the myometrium becomes hypotonic and contractions have greater amplitude. Manipulative treatment, therefore, will be most effective during the week following the end of the period.

When evaluating the results of treatment, be sure to see the patient again at the same point in the hormonal cycle. Uterine movements are under the control of complex central nervous and endocrine factors which can alter tonus, vascular pressure, and cellular fluid absorption. The cervix may open for 1-3 days during ovulation, particularly in a nullipara.

### Intercourse

The movements of the vagina and uterus during intercourse were described by Masters and Johnson (Kolodny, Masters, and Johnson, 1979). During the excitation phase, the superior two-thirds of the vagina becomes oval in shape and increases in volume. During the second phase, the inferior one-third of the vagina contracts. During the third phase (orgasm), there is a rhythmic lifting of the uterus and opening of the cervix. Absence of these movements would inhibit the afferent reflex phenomena and their central stimuli. Lack of proper motion also adversely affects fertility, because of failure of the cervix to open and weak vertical movements of the uterus.

### Pregnancy and Childbirth

During pregnancy, obviously, the uterus increases tremendously in weight and volume. During childbirth there is, in addition, considerable movement and muscular contraction of the uterus. All the uterine ligaments are distended, sometimes to four times their normal length *(Illustration 3-6)*.

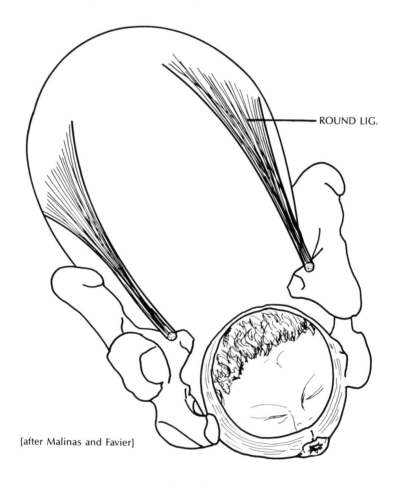

ROUND LIG.

[after Malinas and Favier]

**Illustration 3-6**
Stretching of Ligaments in Pregnancy

You can imagine the problems that a restriction to uterine motion would cause during pregnancy. A locally fixed uterus fibroses around the restriction, presumably leading to reduction in local circulation. We have no definitive proof that the fetus is harmed in these situations, but we prefer not to take the chance.

We have tested partially fixed uteruses in pregnant patients without their knowledge (we did not wish to alarm them needlessly). Nearly all of them remarked near the end of the pregnancy that they felt pain in the exact areas of the restrictions. Sometimes these pains became intense at childbirth.

The uterus must remain mobile in order to efficiently perform its many functions. If none of its attachments are restricted, the uterus moves constantly. During a pelvic examination, do not become unduly concerned about the particular position in which you find the uterus. As long as it is mobile, it is probably functional.

## Normal and Abnormal Anatomy

In the average woman, the uterus makes a 60° angle with the umbilicococcygeal axis, and the angle between the fundus and cervix is 110°–130° *(Illustration 3-7)*. Variations in these angles can result from age, structural type, childbirth, heredity, and numerous diseases which affect uterine attachments and tonus. The curvature of the lumbar spine (lordosis) will always affect the angles of the uterus.

In this section, we will describe some common positional abnormalities. We should note that not all authors use the terms "version" and "flexion" in the same way. In this book,

- *version* is the movement of the uterine body relative to the axis of the pelvis;
- *flexion* is the angle the body forms with the isthmus and cervix.

We also use the terms "anteposition" and "retroposition" of the cervix *(Illustration 3-8)* to refer to its position relative to the pelvis:

- *anteposition* is movement of the cervix toward the symphysis;
- *retroposition* is its movement toward the sacrum.

"Retroflexion" is not synonymous with "retroposition." That is, with a retroflexed uterus, the cervix does not necessarily move closer to the sacrum.

### POSITIONAL ABNORMALITIES

When a nulliparous women (rectum and bladder empty) stands, the cervix, isthmus, and fundus are anteflexed and anteverted. The uterine fundus is several centimeters from the symphysis, and the cervix presses against the posterior vaginal wall, which is thickened at this level.

- The round and uterosacral ligaments sagittally orient and support the uterus.
- The broad ligaments and parametrium restrict sidebending.
- The pelvic subperitoneal tissue and fibrous apparatus of the hypogastric sheath anchor the supravaginal portion of the cervix and the vaginal dome.
- The levator ani and perineum support the pelvic organs.
- Diaphragmatic attraction lessens the effect of gravity and effective weight of the uterus.

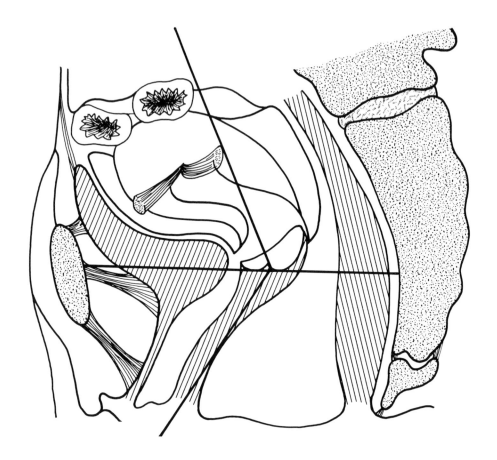

**Illustration 3-7**
Normal Angles of the Uterus

- The combined propulsive and aspirational forces of the cardiovascular system also reduce the effective weight of the uterus.
- The turgor effect facilitates harmonious sliding of the pelvic organs on each other.

## Lateral Deviation

These are often the sequelae of an inflammatory lesion of the pelvis or peritoneum, the fundus being drawn toward the side of the lesion. An ipsilateral ovarian tumor is another possible cause. Congenital sidebending may be due to shortness of a round ligament or to insufficient development of Müller's duct on one side.

Lateral deviations may lead to fibrosis or soft tissue adhesions, which in turn can cause impaired fertility or genital pain. You should check the abdominal peritoneum carefully, because it plays an important role in these restrictions.

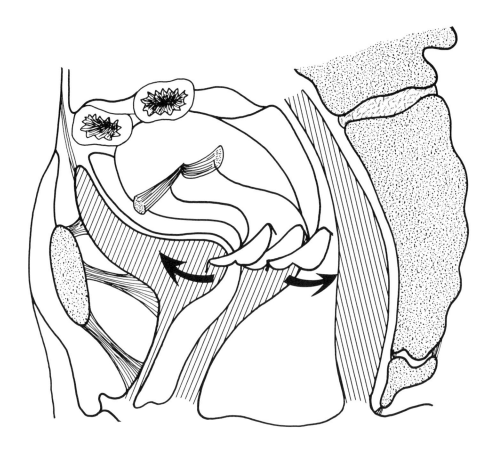

**Illustration 3-8**
Anteposition and Retroposition of the Cervix

## Anterior Deviation

These are less frequent than lateral deviations. They may be congenital (usually due to hypoplasia) or acquired following childbirth or genital infections. Restrictions of the posterior parametrium cause the uterine body to swing forward because of posterosuperior traction of the cervix, posterior vaginal wall, and uterosacral ligaments *(Illustration 3-9)*.

Abnormal tensions in this situation can lead to dysmenorrhea, infertility, bladder irritability (because of direct parietal stimulation), and uterine prolapse. The uterus transmits all abdominal pressures to its anterior aspect and the bladder. Prolapse is usually preceded by verticalization of the uterus.

## Posterior Deviation

Certain weaknesses of the anterior attachment system can be associated with uterine hypoplasia, exaggerated depth of the rectouterine pouch, and collapse of the

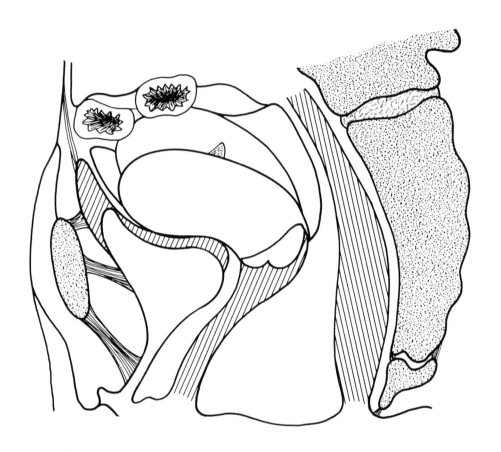

**Illustration 3-9**
Anterior Deviation with Uterine Anteversion

uterus at the back (primary posterior deviation). There may also be hypotonia of the round ligaments, or weakness of the uterovesical wall, pubovesical, or pubo-urethral ligaments.

Secondary posterior deviation has many possible causes:

- Leiomyomas, ovarian cysts, cysts of the broad ligament, or any neoplastic formation in front of the uterus can push it posteriorly.
- Scarring from adnexal lesions pulls the uterus posteriorly. Such scarring, and loss of elasticity of neighboring tissues behind the uterine axis, can retrovert the uterus.
- Tissue infiltration from endometriosis, depending upon its position, can pull the uterus back.
- After surgery, the uterus may stick to the posterior side of the deperitonized broad ligament. In a patient who has undergone *any* type of abdominal or pelvic surgery, you should always assume that there has been an adverse effect on pelvic organ function.

- Pregnancy alters the suspension mechanism of the uterus and brings the isthmus anteroinferiorly. When the uterus does not completely swing toward the back, the vaginal dome prolapses. There may be painful uterine retroversion.
- After motor vehicle accidents, direct hits, or falls on the lumbar area, you may observe retroversion due not to the trauma *per se* but to subsequent scarring. Effects of trauma will be discussed later in this chapter.

The term "**Masters and Allen syndrome**" has been used to describe a combination of obstetrical trauma, uterine retroversion on an over-mobile cervix, and tearing of the posterior and subperitoneal fascia of the broad ligament. This syndrome may arise following childbirth which is too quick or too slow, or application of forceps or suction which tears the cervix, perineum, or cardinal ligaments *(Illustration 3-10)*. It results in restriction of the structures supporting the cervix and isthmus; in particular, the uterosacral ligaments. Pain is low, median and posterior, with a sense of heaviness. Pain is increased by sitting for prolonged periods (tension of the sacrospinous and sacrotuberous ligaments and certain pelvitrochanteric muscles), by fatigue, and by effort. Other symptoms include dysmenorrhea, premenstrual syndrome, and pain on deep penetration and orgasm. Symptoms are relieved by rest in the prone position.

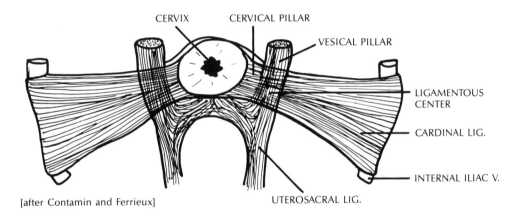

[after Contamin and Ferrieux]

**Illustration 3-10**
Cardinal Ligaments

# CERVIX

## Lengthening of Cervix

If the suspensory structures of the cervix lose their normal tone, one sees hypertrophy and lengthening of the intravaginal portion of the cervix (especially the anterior aspect). Any abdominopelvic pressure will push it downward, since there is nothing to prevent this movement. Lengthening of the cervix occurs only if the rest of the uterus remains well suspended.

## Position of Cervix

On the average, the uterus and cervix form an angle of approximately 110°, but this can vary depending on many factors. The cervix can lengthen and move downward as mentioned above but, more importantly, it can move on a sagittal plane. There are also sidebending, rotation, and combinations of these movements. Our experience has shown that two positions, anteposition and retroposition (see Illustration 3-8) are particularly pathogenic. In anteposition, the cervix is fixed anteriorly and slightly superiorly, and presses on the bladder neck/trigonal region via the anterior vaginal wall. The resulting irritation can lead to incontinence, especially during the premenstrual period. Intercourse in the prone position is painful and can provoke the urge to urinate.

In retroposition, the cervix is fixed posteriorly, and presses against the rectum via the posterior vaginal septum and rectouterine pouch. This leads to reflex constipation, tenesmus, and hemorrhoidal premenstrual pressure.

Retroversion of the uterus usually means anteposition of the cervix, while anteversion of the uterus can be associated with ante- or retroposition of the cervix. The position of the cervix is of greater concern than that of the uterus. A retroverted uterus which is fully mobile rarely poses a significant problem.

## Ptosis and Prolapse

Ptosis is the initial stage of a prolapse. A prolapse is a serious distention or even outright rupture of the means of attachment of the uterus or other organ (Illustration 3-11). Ptoses and prolapses result from failure of suspensory and support structures, and can be primary or secondary. Primary causes are anomalies of the axial curvature of the pelvis, and muscular hypoplasia. Secondary causes are obstetrical trauma, surgery, postmenopausal involution, etc.

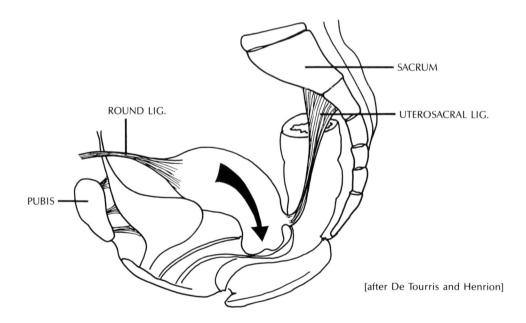

SACRUM

ROUND LIG.

UTEROSACRAL LIG.

PUBIS

[after De Tourris and Henrion]

**Illustration 3-11**
Uterine Prolapse

According to Lansac and Lecompte (1981), prolapses include "all permanent protrusions, with effort, in the vaginal lumen, the vulval orifice or, apart from this, all or one part of the vaginal walls more or less doubled by the bladder, the rectum and the adjacent peritoneal pouches, as well as the solid vaginal bottom of the cervix."

Some prolapses are difficult to detect clinically and are more pronounced at a certain stage of the menstrual cycle. If more practitioners did a more thorough job of taking the history and doing the physical examination, there would be less hasty and uncalled for classification of patients as belonging to the categories of hystrionic or hysterical neurosis.[1] This is because, before a prolapse sets in, the tissues must already have been injured. These injuries cause problems or restrictions which are more or less apparent depending upon the cycle and the general condition of the patient. A ptosis is even more discreet in its symptomatology and only a careful and intensive examination can uncover it. On top of this, it can be labile depending upon the moment of the day, general constitution, and stage of the menstrual cycle.

PTOSIS: This typically means a slight relaxing of the support structures of the uterus, which still retains its general shape. A prolapse does not just happen spontaneously; the tissues must already have been injured or predisposed to injury in some way. Ptoses are harder to detect than prolapses, and their manifestation can depend on health of the individual, time of day, or stage of menstrual cycle.

CLASSIFICATION OF PROLAPSES: Naming depends on position. For prolapses of the vagina:

- urethrocele = urethral segment;
- anterior colpocele = vesical segment (also known as cystourethrocele);
- elytrocele = rectouterine pouch segment (also known as elytrocele; see below);
- posterior colpocele = rectal segment (also known as rectocele).

For prolapses of the uterus:

- 1st degree = cervix is intravaginal;
- 2nd degree = cervix is level with vulva;
- 3rd degree = cervix is outside vulvar orifice.

## Elytrocele

In this posterior vaginal hernia, the rectouterine pouch descends (through the rectovaginal septum), between the levators, and ends up on the perineal body. The pressure from the elytrocele increases uterine prolapse, the peritoneum is brought along by the unwinding of the vagina, and the small intestine infiltrates between the vagina and rectum in the rectouterine pouch (Illustration 3-12). Elytrocele is often associated with uterine prolapse or retroversion.

With retroversion, the uterus obliterates the rectouterine pouch by taking its place. It tends to push itself between the levators under abdominopelvic pressure. This is often seen as a sequela to hysteropexy. When the vertical mobility of the uterus is exaggerated, the posterior vagina unwinds along with its peritoneal covering.

---

1. It is interesting to note that "hysteria" is the Greek for "a uterine condition." This demonstrates the bias inherent in this term and its use against women.

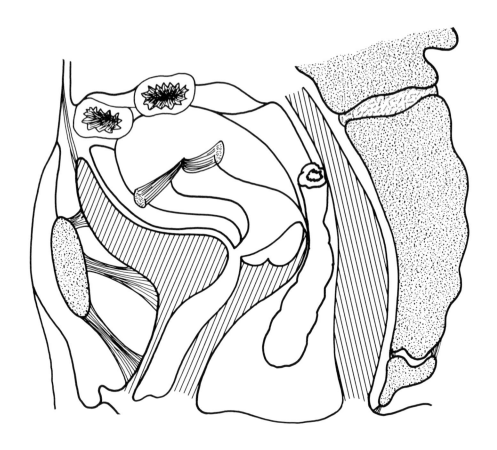

**Illustration 3-12**
Elytrocele

Normal distribution of intracavitary pressures and fluid circulation requires that all pelvic organs have normal relations to one another. If the uterus is retroverted, abdominal pressures will tend to push it inferoposteriorly. Compression of the vascular system results in accumulation of venous and lymphatic fluid, increasing the weight of the uterus and decreasing the effects of abdominal suction. This vicious cycle moves the uterus even further posteriorly and hastens its evolution toward ptosis or prolapse.

## Articular Physiology

The articular physiology of this area is incredibly complex. In fact, it would take an entire book to describe it. In this section we will be satisfied to briefly describe the pelvic articulations. We hope that this emphasis will enable you to comprehend and visualize the extent of the interdependence between the skeletal system and pelvic organs.

## Directions and Planes

The human pelvis differ from that of anthropoid apes in several important ways. The human sacrum is longer and not parallel to the pubic symphysis, the sacral promontory is closer to the pubis, and the pelvic cavity is shorter from top to bottom. This means that the vulval orifice is in front of the fetal track. In addition, because of the obliqueness of the sacrum:

- the anal orifice is higher than the vulval orifice;
- the vulva faces anteroinferiorly, which is different from the direction in which the uterus pushes the fetus;
- the pelvic inlet is the space between the sacral promontory and pubis;
- the pelvic outlet is the space between the ischiopubic rami and coccyx.

The plane of least dimensions (also known as the middle strait) is found between the inferior edge of the pubis and the sciatic spine *(Illustration 3-13)*. The dimensions of this plane are smaller than those of other planes within the pelvic cavity. It is enlarged with extension of the sacrum.

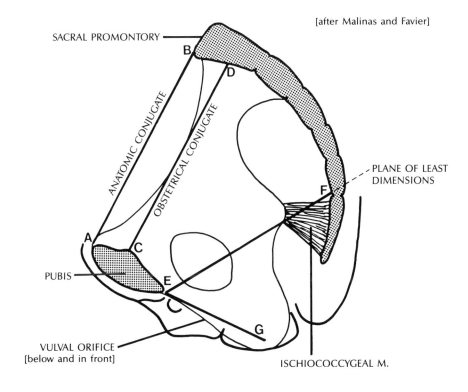

**Illustration 3-13**
Obstetrical Planes

### Pelvic Cavity

The volume of the pelvic cavity in non-pregnant women is 800-900ml. That of the fetal head is of 500-600ml. This makes the cavity big enough for any diameter of fetal head to pass, except for the verticomental.

Mobility of the pelvis is still crucial. The pelvis is usually mobile enough to assure easy passage of the fetus. Exceptions are due to such osseous non-articular pathological conditions as sequelae of rickets, significant pelvic asymmetries, hip dislocations, Pott's disease, and pelvic fractures. Good overall pelvic mobility requires satisfactory movement of the sacroiliac and sacrococcygeal joints, ischiatic separation, and painless mobility of the lumbar vertebra.

### Sacrum

Movements of the sacrum often have greater amplitude than described in conventional gynecological texts, where, for example, anterior flexion ("nutation") is given as 2mm. When the sacrum flexes, the sagittal diameter of the plane of least dimensions increases by at least a centimeter, making it more than 12cm *(Illustration 3-14)*. This causes lowering of the uterus and changes the axes of the various pelvic planes.

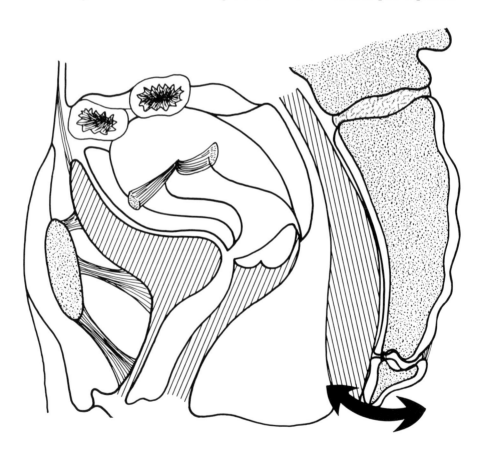

**Illustration 3-14**
Sacral Flexion

Flexion or adduction of the thighs causes the adductors and other thigh muscles which originate from the ischium to contract and become tense. The ilia move on the sacrum, the pubis moves upward, the promontory-symphysis distance lessens, and the plane of least dimensions becomes nearly vertical, converging with the axis along which the uterus is lowered.

## Lumbosacral Angle

Some gynecologists take this angle into consideration in estimating the possibility or progress of dystocia (abnormal labor). However, imaging techniques frequently show a "pathological" angle, and subsequent childbirth is problem-free. This is another example of a positional factor without great importance. We prefer testing the *mobility* of L5-S1.

## Ischiatic Separation

This can be evaluated by radiography or by manual examination, which we prefer. We caution against making any obstetrical prognosis based solely on a simple bi-ischiatic radiometric measure. This is because when someone gets up after sitting down the ischia move apart by more than one centimeter. Anytime a person rises from a sitting position, the ischia move apart by more than one centimeter.

Our major concern is that the ischia should be mobile in order to facilitate functioning of the pelvis. This requires good elasticity of the sacrospinous and sacrotuberous ligaments, coccygeus muscles, levators, perineal body, and pelvitrochanteric muscles.

## Sacrococcygeal Joint

The sacrococcygeal angle should increase with abdominal pressure (e.g., pushing efforts, defecation, childbirth, seated position), and decrease with contraction of the perineum. This angle is smaller in standing than in sitting position. The anterior-posterior movement has an amplitude of approximately 30°. Fixation of the sacrococcygeal joint interferes with normal childbirth and may necessitate use of suction or forceps.

## Lumbar and Sacroiliac Joints

For the ischia to move apart, the ilia must get closer to the median sacral axis and L5 must undergo anterior flexion. These combined movements should have good amplitude and be totally painless. Routine lower back pain can become intolerable during childbirth and interfere with normal delivery. For this reason, it is essential to maintain good elasticity of the many ligaments of the lumbar and sacroiliac regions. These include the iliolumbar, interspinal, supraspinal, sacrotuberous, and sacrospinous. You should familiarize yourself with the tests for all of these.

Many gynecologists now recognize that the sacroiliac joints, far from being fixed or immobile, have a central reflexogenic effect through their mechanoreceptors. This effect helps promote normal childbirth.

## Presentation of Fetus

Among all mammals, the human fetus is the only one whose head cannot fit through the sagittal diameter of the pelvis, because of projection of the sacral promontory. During presentation, the more the head of the fetus is flexed, the smaller is the diameter of engagement. The largest diameter is the biparietal (distance between the two parietal eminences). When the sacrum is only slightly concave and cannot be mobilized, the cylinder of engagement is reduced in volume, which makes passage of the head more difficult.

*It is therefore better to have a reduced pelvic inlet and a concave and mobilizable sacrum, than a large inlet with a flat and fixed sacrum.*

The anus separates the anterior from the posterior perineum and is midway between the two ischia. During childbirth, the perineum swings posteriorly. The fetus presses against the anus or perineal body, but never against the vulva *(Illustration 3-15)*.

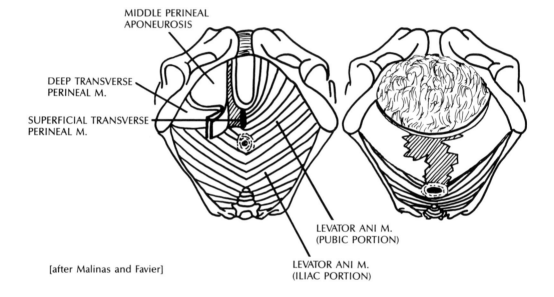

MIDDLE PERINEAL APONEUROSIS

DEEP TRANSVERSE PERINEAL M.

SUPERFICIAL TRANSVERSE PERINEAL M.

LEVATOR ANI M. (PUBIC PORTION)

[after Malinas and Favier]

LEVATOR ANI M. (ILIAC PORTION)

**Illustration 3-15**
Presentation of Fetus

The deepest and most resistant part of the perineal body is behind the vagina, and consists of interlaced fibers of the elevator fasciculi of the levator ani, between the pubis and anus. During childbirth, this portion is pushed downward, compressed between the fetal head and perineum. The muscles are distended and squashed, and the anal sphincter becomes a slim ring. With extension of the head, the pressure imposed on the muscles increases and divides them into isolated and flattened fasciculi.

The fibers of the levator ani become dissociated around the head. There are small hematomas and tears, followed later by scarring and replacement of muscle by fibrous tissue. This functional loss is aggravated by pulling of the levators (particularly the median fibers) out of their insertions, so that they retain only their sphincteral attachments. Connective tissue structures such as the vesicovaginal fascia also suffer from these mechanical stresses.

As the fetus moves further downward, it presses against the coccyx and pushes it posteriorly. The anococcygeal body elongates and the retroanal region bulges. Anovulval distance triples or even quadruples. The vulva orients itself anteriorly. During the period of intense stretching, the sacrococcygeal joint, anococcygeal body, and middle perineal aponeurosis often undergo trauma. In multiparas, the middle perineal aponeurosis which surrounds the vulva always presents some torn or distended fibers. In nulliparas, the uterosacral ligaments help suspend the uterus from the sacrum in a standing position. With vaginal childbirth, these ligaments are often torn and later replaced by useless fibrous tissue. This is even more prevalent with meaningless obstetrical maneuvers, especially when they are not coordinated with bearing down efforts.

## PATHOLOGY

### Pelvic Articulations

In comparison with the well-known tests of the vertebral column, those of the pelvic articulations are too often neglected. The bony pelvis is a massive structure requiring powerful ligaments for stabilization. The elasticity of these ligaments is extremely important. Loss of this elasticity (e.g., because of pregnancy, childbirth, sedentary occupation, trauma, aging) prevents anterior flexion of the sacrum; the body compensates for this through increased movement of the lower lumbar vertebrae. This leads to excessive wear and eventual erosion of the intervertebral discs.

A fixed pelvis will adversely affect childbirth, pregnancy, and mobility of the urogenital organs. A pelvic restriction always changes the normal axes of movement, and redirects intrapelvic pressures.

The muscles and ligaments of the pelvic joints are very reflexogenic, and affect functioning of urogenital structures through hypothalamic stimulation. Fibrosis or other restrictions can prevent the afferent tracts from sending messages to the cortex. Sometimes 1cm of movement of the sacrum may be the difference between eutocia and dystocia. This demonstrates what an important preventative role osteopathy can play in obstetrics.

### Intrapelvic Soft Tissues

Soft tissues tend to lose their elasticity through chronic mechanical tension. Imagine an adhesion of the left uterosacral ligament. Each time that the subject walks, breathes, has sex, has a full bladder or rectum, is premenstrual, etc., the anterior-posterior movement of the uterus takes place on a modified axis, with a sidebending rotation. Gradually, the uterus rests on its side and compresses its vascular system. It becomes edematous and heavy, pulling on its supporting muscle or connective fibers until they are stretched or damaged. Retroversion, ptosis, or prolapse can easily follow.

The importance of reciprocal tensions in pelvic function was discussed in chapter 1. A fixed organ tends to pull other organs toward itself. Typically, the sacrogenital folds and uterosacral ligaments contract and the pelvis becomes very painful. If fluid circulation is deficient, the organs are vulnerable to the numerous pathogenic agents which constantly surround them. Urogenital manipulation has aims other than normalization of intrapelvic mobility; it also helps re-establish normal fluid circulation and immune function. Fibrosis brings about mechanical stretching of nerve fibers, whose chronic stimulation causes the vasomotor and muscular systems to go into spasm. The pelvic ligaments are all contractile and highly interdependent.

Normally, movement between the various organs is facilitated by the presence of serous fluid (e.g., in the rectouterine pouch). With inflammatory conditions, the connective organization of fibrinous exudate can actually create capsules, septa, or bands which isolate or encapsulate the organs. Surface adhesions can join the deep side of the ovary to the broad ligament and edge of the uterus, or join the uterine tube to the base of the ovary.

# Indications for Treatment

## Lower Back Pain

Most osteopaths see their primary role as testing and correcting vertebral restrictions. However, if a fixed sacrum is secondary to a uterine retroversion, every time the sacrum is released it will soon return to its restricted state. In this case, the uterus must be released before the sacrum is manipulated. Cases of lower back pain often result from urogenital restrictions. If the lower back pain is aggravated in the seated position and accompanied by sensations of gastric and rectal congestion, it is probably due to a sacrococcygeal joint problem. Visceral restrictions can be secondary to osteoarticular restrictions, but the reverse situation is more common. Later in this chapter, we will describe tests that enable you to differentiate between primary visceral and primary osteoarticular restrictions.

## Adhesions

Pelvic adhesions are common sequelae of surgery, infection, trauma, childbirth, etc. They inevitably affect the static and dynamic relationships of the pelvic cavity and the organs it contains. Anytime you encounter an adhesion or scar you must carefully evaluate its effects.

The list of *infectious agents* capable of attacking urogenital organs and structures is very long. Infection often leads to scarring, which carries the risk of serious consequences such as occlusion of the uterine tubes.

Common types of *trauma* affecting the abdomen and pelvis are direct impact, falls, gunshots, knife wounds, and motor vehicle accidents.

*Childbirth*, even without complications, is already an ordeal for the pelvic tissues—an ordeal which is considerably worsened by heavy-handed obstetrical techniques. Let us make it clear that we are not at all for a return to the primitive conditions whereby women gave birth on the run between domestic duties. Too many women and children have lost their lives under those conditions. But why, when childbirth is taking place satisfactorily, use suction or a large episiotomy? Why stimulate contractions? Why infiltrate the pudendal nerve? Why use epidural anesthesia? Do obstetricians consider all the consequences of these interventions? Why not tilt the delivery table closer to the vertical, and take advantage of gravity? Although this may not be a very glamorous comparison, it is not easy to defecate while lying down on the toilet. In our opinion, obstetrical intervention should be used only in cases of clear dystocia. This would help both mothers and babies avoid many subsequent problems.

## Stability Problems

Static problems are those that are related to the stability of the reproductive organs. They are usually associated with those of the urinary organs and vary greatly with age and medical history. You should worry less about putting a structure "back in its place" than about restoring its mobility and elasticity. Sometimes a uterus will always be retroverted in spite of anything we may do.

Static problems range from simple, localized restrictions to ptoses and prolapses. We can often help with first or second degree uterine prolapses, but seldom with third degree prolapses.

## Dyspareunia and Anorgasmia

Dyspareunia arising from vesical problems was discussed in chapter 2. Structural problems of the uterus or vagina (restriction, ptosis, or prolapse) can also make intercourse difficult and painful. Of course, anorgasmia and loss of libido can also have psychological or emotional origins. But be careful to rule out physical explanations first.

## Circulatory Problems

Restriction or ptosis of the uterus can disturb arterial, venous, and lymphatic circulation of the pelvis and lower extremities. This occurs through both direct compression and reflex vascular spasms. A retroverted, non-mobile uterus is often purplish-blue in color, edematous, and heavy. When a surgeon verticalizes it and normal circulation is restored, it quickly recovers its normal pinkish color.

## Infertility

It is difficult to say definitively whether osteopathic manipulation can resolve cases of infertility. The factors affecting fertility (psychological, relational, hormonal, climatic, etc.) are complex and poorly understood. Certainly our manipulations can improve the mobility of ovaries, uterine tubes, and uterus, which presumably increases the chances that egg and sperm will meet under favorable conditions. We strongly believe that osteopathic treatment locally stimulates the pelvic organs, afferent nerve fibers, and hypothalamic-pituitary axis. We have been able to objectively demonstrate our effects on tubular mobility, but *not* on the hypothalamus. We have had four similar cases of patients married for more than five years, not using any contraceptive device, and apparently unable to conceive. In each case, the patient became pregnant after osteopathic treatment for lower back pain, although we had never mentioned possible effects on fertility. Anecdotal evidence like this is suggestive, but does not prove a cause-and-effect relationship.

## Dysmenorrhea and Pelvic Pain

This is a complicated subject, since menstrual and other pelvic pains can have many causes. In general, osteopathic treatment can relieve these types of pain when there is an articular or visceral mechanical cause. As mentioned earlier, with chronic restrictions local nervous feedback to the central nervous system decreases. This disturbs the feedback loop so that, to some extent, the local area ceases to "be there" to the central nervous system. This in turn decreases the efferent information going to the area. We believe that manipulation can break this vicious cycle, and that our long-term effects are often related to this phenomenon.

### Prevention of Obstetrical Problems

This is as important for the nullipara as for the multipara. Gestation and child-birth can be complicated by a variety of factors. A sacroiliac restriction can inhibit certain pelvic mechanical reflexes which are indispensable for smooth labor and delivery. When you encounter problems in a multipara, look for a structural cause. With a nullipara, test the osteoarticular and visceral systems from a preventative point of view.

# *Mobility Tests*

## PELVIC OSTEOARTICULAR SYSTEM

It is frustrating to see an osteopathic treatment fail because of an undiagnosed joint dysfunction. Before undertaking pelvic visceral treatment, you should test the mechanics of the following joints:

- lumbar spine
- lumbosacral
- sacroiliac
- sacrococcygeal
- pubic symphysis
- sacrotuberous
- hip.

Tests of some joints (e.g., symphysis, ischial) may be less familiar to you than others. For all pelvic joints, "bent knee" testing is usually most appropriate. For this, you are behind the standing patient. Place a thumb on each posterosuperior iliac spine (PSIS) and ask the patient to bend one knee at a time, over and over. This test allows you to evaluate the mobility of the sacroiliac joints at all levels (superior, middle, inferior). Tests of the sacrum and coccyx, which have close connections with the uterine attachment system, will be described later.

## EXTERNAL ROUTE

### Small Intestine and Greater Omentum

These structures should be tested before you specifically examine the reproductive organs. With a lower restriction of the small intestine, pressure is exerted upon the uterine fundus on an abnormal axis. The small intestine can infiltrate in front of or behind the uterus, especially when the rectum and bladder are empty. Sometimes the small intestine may actually become fixed in these areas.

SUPINE POSITION: Slightly raise the patient's pelvis on a cushion to free the small intestine, and explore the abdomen following lines directed toward the umbilicus. Find the root of the mesentery, a cord-like structure extending from the cecum to the area below the duodenojejunal junction. Gently push your fingers well in and stretch the fibers on either side of the root until it is all released.

LEFT LATERAL DECUBITUS POSITION: This position makes it relatively easy to explore the abdominopelvic region, especially the low infiltrations of the small intestine. Place your fingers in the iliac fossa. Push them first posteriorly and pedad deeper into the pelvis; then bring them anteriorly and toward the umbilicus *(Illustration 3-16)*. In this way you can evaluate the anterior parietal peritoneum. Any injury to this structure, even high in the abdomen, can affect the whole system of cavitary pressures. One cannot perceive a healthy peritoneum by palpation, but its injury following trauma, surgery, or infection makes it hard, fibrous, sclerosed and therefore palpable.

## Median and Medial Umbilical Ligaments

These tests were mentioned in chapter 2, and are also useful for the uterus. Restriction of these ligaments typically leads to anterior restriction of the uterus. The tests can be done in various positions: seated, supine, or lateral decubitus. Place your fingers on the line going from the umbilicus to the symphysis. You can then evaluate the distensibility of the median umbilical ligament on the medial line *(Illustration 3-17)*. The medial umbilical ligaments are on two oblique lines running from the umbilicus to areas near the medial iliopubic rami. Place your fingers on these two lines, near their insertions on the rami. To test the elasticity of the tissues, press your fingers posteriorly and then both medially and laterally.

## Uterine Fundus

The peritoneum can be disengaged from the cervix but is always closely attached to the fundus. The suspensory role of the peritoneum is demonstrated by the phenomenon of reciprocal tension which orients the uterus. Restrictions of the peritoneum can restrict the uterus, and bring it into rotation or sidebending depending on its position. The fundus is usually located at the level of the bladder, behind the iliopubic rami. Approach it via the lateral edge of the rectus abdominis, or, if present, via a diastasis of the linea alba. Direct your fingers first laterally, then posteriorly, and only then toward the median axis. Make the tissues play upon the fundus by stretching them. A restriction will manifest itself by scarring, pain, or poor tissue distensibility.

This external test lets you evaluate the upper part of the anterior uterine pouch, and possible involvement of the bladder, sigmoid colon, and rectum in a uterine problem. When the uterus is retroverted, your fingers do not press on the fundus during this test. However, their pressure in the direction of the sacrum provokes pain (sometimes quite intense) which confirms the abnormal position of the uterus. In order to facilitate deep exploration, work with one hand and then the other, and bring the patient's knees (one or both) toward the thorax. The more the thighs are flexed, the more accessible the deeper pelvic structures.

## Round Ligaments

These fibromuscular cords are almost impossible to identify precisely by palpation, yet their restriction adversely affects uterine orientation and support. An injury to one ligament brings the uterus into sidebending and rotation. If both are injured, the uterus remains pressed forward. Again, it is not the position which is pathological, but the loss of mobility. A common problem secondary to round ligament restriction is the inability of the uterus to verticalize with pushing by the bladder.

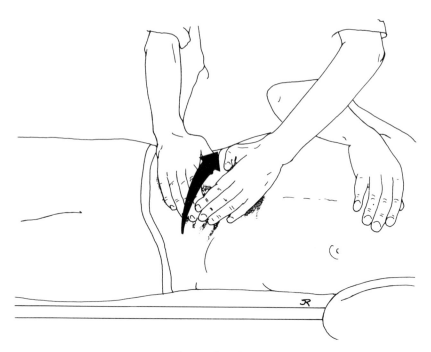

**Illustration 3-16**
Small Intestine Test: Left Lateral Decubitus Position

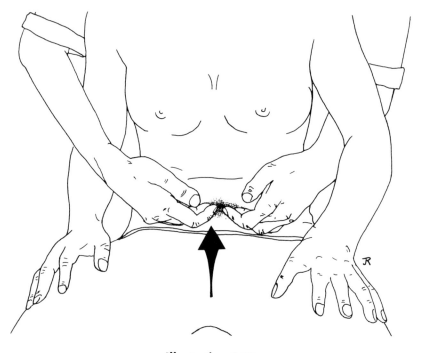

**Illustration 3-17**
Median Umbilical Ligament Test

Because it is so difficult to palpate the round ligaments, you should be familiar with their location and insertion *(Illustration 3-18)*. The insertion sites are:

- anterolateral uterus;
- inguinal canal, where they send fibers in many directions;
- pubic spine and anterior symphysis.

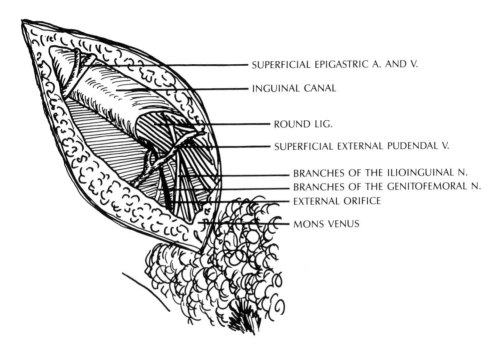

SUPERFICIAL EPIGASTRIC A. AND V.

INGUINAL CANAL

ROUND LIG.

SUPERFICIAL EXTERNAL PUDENDAL V.

BRANCHES OF THE ILIOINGUINAL N.
BRANCHES OF THE GENITOFEMORAL N.
EXTERNAL ORIFICE

MONS VENUS

**Illustration 3-18**
External Insertion of the Round Ligament

The ligament is tested with the patient in supine position, legs bent. Place your fingers on the external inguinal canals and gently stretch the ligaments by moving your fingers transversely back and forth. Evaluate the elasticity of the tissues and compare the left and right sides to see if either is restricted. The test is positive if you feel sensitive fibrous tissues, and if the uterus is fixed in a position of anterior flexion or sidebending rotation on the sclerosed side. Skill in this test requires considerable practice.

The round ligament, in the fold of the groin, is accompanied by the genital branches of the genitofemoral and the ilioinguinal nerves. Naturally, fibrosis of the ligament affects function of these nerves.

### Pubovesical Ligaments

Elasticity of these ligaments is important for normal sliding of the pelvic organs during active movements (pushing) or passive movements (walking, breathing, physical exercise). The ligaments are connected to the pillars of the bladder, which help join the cervix to the bladder. Therefore, restriction of these ligaments affects the uterus.

To test the pubovesicals, press your fingers against the posterior part of the symphysis and direct them inferiorly. Approach from the sides in order to get around and partially avoid the anterior abdominal attachments. Flex the thighs toward the thorax and evaluate the elasticity of the ligaments by wiggling the finger under the pubis (*Illustration 3-19*). Different positions are possible; see chapter 2 for details.

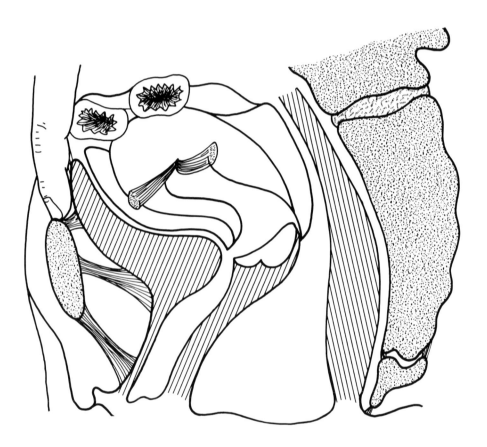

**Illustration 3-19**
Pubovesical Ligament Test

## Broad Ligaments

These are peritoneal folds that change position depending on the volume of the bladder and state of the uterus. They should be relatively easy to mobilize. Their thin superior and lateral portions are accessible but difficult to distinguish from surrounding tissues. A unilateral restriction of the broad ligament brings the uterus into ipsilateral sidebending. A bilateral restriction fixes the uterus in high retroversion, with less cervical retroflexion and retroposition than occurs with a uterosacral restriction. These ligaments can be tested in various positions, as described below. They will be discussed again in chapter 4.

LATERAL DECUBITUS POSITION: Stand posterior to the patient to test the ligament on the side nearest the table. Place your fingers inside the anterosuperior iliac spine (A.S.I.S.) and then move them posteriorly and slightly inferiorly. Leave the fingers against the ilium at first so that you can, gradually, move them deeply and medially toward the uterus *(Illustration 3-20)*. Otherwise, you will soon be on the intestine instead of the broad ligament. This test allows you to discover deep micro-adhesions.

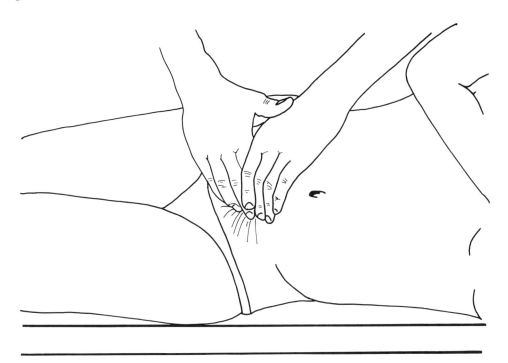

**Illustration 3-20**
Broad Ligament Test: Lateral Decubitus Position

Incidentally, the suspensory ligament of the ovary follows the lateral edge of the broad ligament, lengthens at the top and lateral side of the iliac fossa, crosses the psoas, and inserts on the prelumbar fascia. It is not impossible to find a restriction of this ligament, because it follows the external edge of the broad ligament, lengthens at the top and outside of the iliac fossa, crosses the psoas and ends on the prelumbar fascia. As with the median umbilical ligament, we do not think that we can directly feel it, but its retraction causes a restriction of the broad ligament. In this manner we can indirectly sense its restrictions through the effects it has on the broad ligament.

MODIFIED TRENDELENBURG POSITION: You are seated to the side of the examining table. The patient lies with her knees bent, sacrum on the table, and head and shoulders resting on your thighs. Gravity helps remove the pressure of the intestinal mass on the pelvic organs. To release abdominal tension, use one hand to flex the legs. With the other hand, evaluate the elasticity of the broad ligaments *(Illustration 3-21)*. Compare one side with the other.

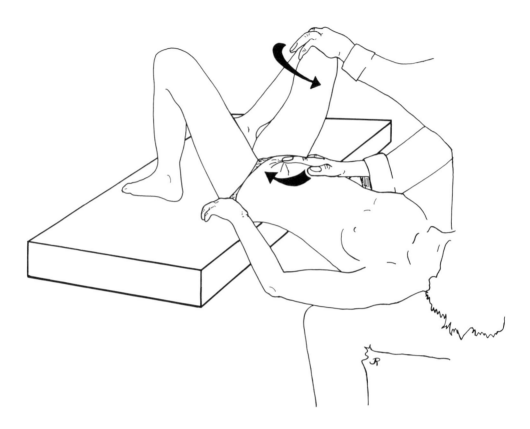

**Illustration 3-21**
Broad Ligament Test: Modified Trendelenburg Position

KNEE/ELBOW POSITION: This position prevents the abdominal muscles from contracting and pushing away your hand. Place your fingers on either side of the inferior part of the lateral edge of the rectus abdominis, or, if there is a diastasis, between the medial edges. Approach the uterus laterally, facing the posterior edge of the symphysis, and test the broad ligaments (*Illustration 3-22*).

In the case of a retroversion, this position has the advantage of bringing the uterus anteriorly and reducing the posterior concavity of the broad ligaments, which increases their accessibility. The pressure of the abdominal organs is no longer from top to bottom but from back to front, which draws the uterus forward. This situation allows you to test the pubovesical and median umbilical ligaments as well.

## Subpubic Region

The perineal body is located between the vulva and anus (see chapter 2). With the patient in supine position, legs bent, push this hard mass superiorly with the thumb (*Illustration 3-23*). If you feel little resistance, or if the perineal body seems flat and dissociated, the perineum is probably hypotonic and distended. This simple technique permits evaluation of the tonicity of the levator ani, voluntary anal sphincter, vaginal constrictors, and superficial and deep transverse perineal muscles. A deficient perineal body requires another test by the rectal route (described later).

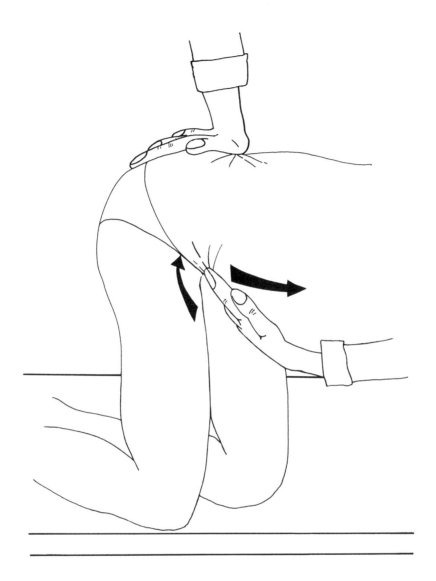

**Illustration 3-22**
Broad Ligament Test: Knee/Elbow Position

## Obturator Region

The obturator test is used primarily in relation to bladder problems. However, obturator restrictions tend to have effects, via the bladder, on the anterior uterus and perineum. The lateral vesical fascia continues as the pubovesical and uterovesical ligaments, which mingle laterally with the pelvic aponeurosis until the sciatic anchorages. This aponeurosis joins the internal obturator, levator ani, and their aponeuroses. Thus, an obturator injury affects the support system of the uterus.

Place the patient in supine position, leg on the tested side bent, the other straight.

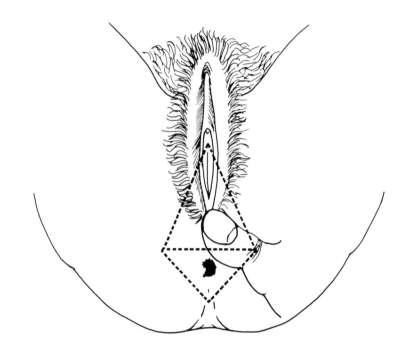

**Illustration 3-23**
Perineal Body Test

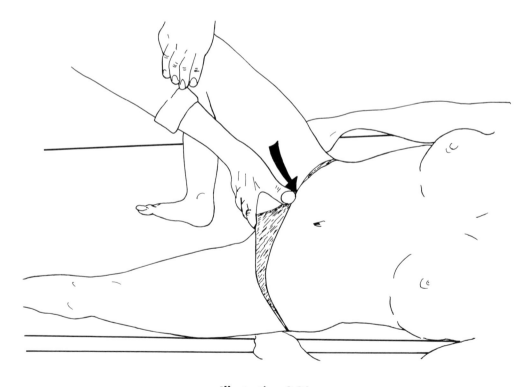

**Illustration 3-24**
Obturator Test

Slide your thumb (rest of hand open) along the adductors until the insertion of the adductor longus and pectineus on the ischiopubic ramus *(Illustration 3-24)*. Move your hand superolaterally and behind the obturator foramen, and test all the neighboring tissues. To increase penetration of your fingers in the obturator foramen, flex and rotate the hip joint, and try utilizing diaphragmatic respiration. For more information on this test, see chapter 2.

### Ischiorectal Fossa

SUPINE POSITION: The patient's legs are bent. Test the two fossae alternately by pressing the pads of the fingers against first the medial edge of the ischium and then the lateral edge of the anus *(Illustration 3-25)*.

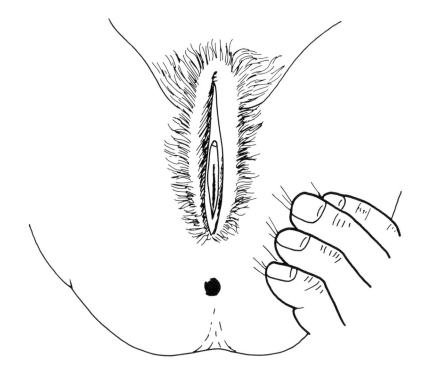

**Illustration 3-25**
Ischiorectal Fossa Test: Supine Position

When against the medial edge of the ischium, your fingers are on the internal obturator and levator ani muscles, along with their aponeuroses. Posteriorly, they are on the coccygeus muscle and sacrospinous ligament. At the sciatic spine, you will feel the coccygeus and levator ani muscles along with the sacrospinous ligament. Move these structures away from the ischium, toward the anus, to check for tears or adhesions. When against the lateral edge of the anus, your fingers are on the levator ani. Anteriorly, they are on the anobulbar raphe; posteriorly, over the anococcygeal body. Stretch these structures to test their elasticity and to check for restrictions.

With effort, the cervix presses against the anococcygeal body similarly to the way the uterus presses against this body during pregnancy. Injuries to this body have serious consequences for uterine function:

- if too weak, the anococcygeal body keeps the cervix in permanent "pushing" position and the uterus moves posteriorly;
- if fibrosed, the body keeps the cervix in permanent retention position and affects the bladder and its attachments.

During this test, one can also examine the pubic insertion of the levators, found 4-5mm above the subpubic ligament.

SEATED POSITION: This test has the advantage of placing the tissues and organs in a position of normal weight distribution, but requires considerable experience and skill for successful interpretation. The patient is sitting, legs unsupported. With one arm, bring the trunk into sidebending so that only one ischium remains on the table. Place the fingers of your free arm against the medial edge of the uplifted ischium, then return the pelvis to normal seated position. In this position, the ischia will be pushed apart. As much as possible, stretch all the tissues directly or indirectly inserted in the ischia, and push the tissues in all possible directions *(Illustration 3-26)*. Other procedures are as described for the supine position.

A perineum which is too easily depressed is hypotonic and slack. Treatment of this problem is relatively difficult. Lateral fixation of the perineum usually reflects zones of adhesion, and is easier to treat.

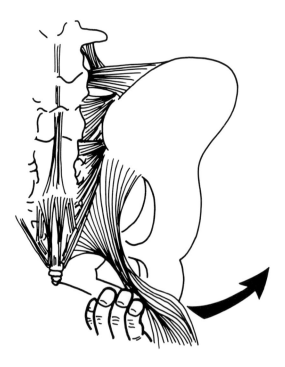

**Illustration 3-26**
Ischiorectal Fossa Test: Seated Position

During the seated test, you can also evaluate the lateral aspects of the sacro-coccygeal joint, by pushing the coccyx to one side. Sensation of pain at the joint indicates an articular restriction. Pain felt between the ischium and coccyx indicates a perineal restriction.

### Sacrum

In chapter 2 (pages 62–63) we described a test of the pubic symphysis, because its restriction can disturb the anterior vesical attachment system. Similarly, a sacral restriction will disturb the uterine attachment system. The sacral test with compression provides information on the posterior uterine attachments, and helps differentiate osteoarticular problems from visceral ones.

Place the subject on her stomach, the anterosuperior iliac spines resting on a cushion. The uterosacral ligaments arise from the isthmus and insert at the level of S2-S4. Place the palm of one hand upon the other and compress the sacrum between the ilia in the direction of the isthmus, pressing upon S2-S4 (Illustration 3-27).

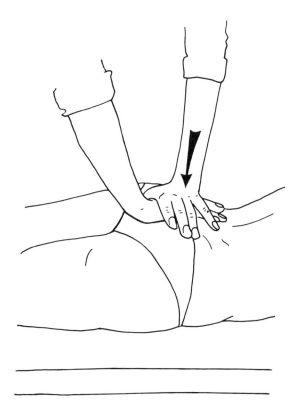

**Illustration 3-27**
Sacral Test with Compression

- If there is a unilateral sacroiliac restriction, movement is immediately blocked, or only the side opposite the restriction moves.

- With bilateral uterosacral restriction, the sacrum is difficult to mobilize and takes a long time returning to its original position. With unilateral uterosacral restriction, the sacrum does not immediately move into sidebending (as with a sacroiliac restriction), but does so during the return movement.

This test requires great skill and sensitivity, and should always be corroborated by lateral tests of the cervix, performed via the internal route.

### Coccyx

Familiarity with this external coccygeal test is essential, since not all patients can be tested via the rectal route. The coccyx can be affected by fibromuscular pelvic problems, and also by direct trauma. Restriction of the coccyx is usually anterior, and sometimes there is an actual anterior subluxation. The sacrococcygeal is one of the rare joints subject to positional restrictions (the others are the chondrocostal, sternocostal, and sterno-clavicular). We prefer testing the coccyx in the seated position because pressure from the abdominopelvic organs and gravity, stretching of the sacrococcygeal and ischiococcygeal ligaments, and ischiatic separation prevent any compensation by other structures in this area.

SEATED POSITION: With one arm, sidebend the patient so that only one ischium remains on the table. Place the free hand on the sacrum and move the index finger toward the coccyx (which is located further anterior than most people think). Return the pelvis to normal sitting position. As the finger moves forward, bend it so that the pad remains

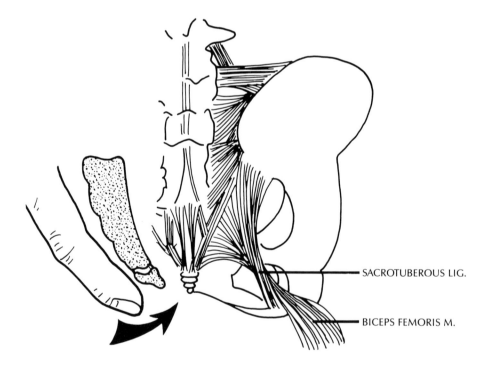

**Illustration 3-28**
Coccygeal Test: Seated Position

in contact with the coccygeal curvature. At the end, push the coccyx superiorly and slightly posteriorly *(Illustration 3-28)*. A fixed joint will cause immediate pain during the pushing. You can also carry out and evaluate backward bending and sidebending of the vertebral column in this position.

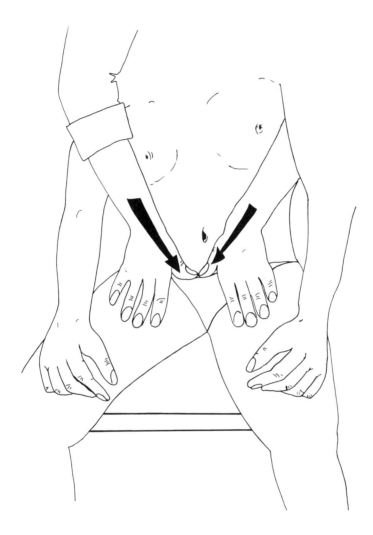

**Illustration 3-29**
Coccygeal Test: Aggravation

AGGRAVATION TEST: This test is useful for confirming positional abnormalities of the uterus, or injuries to its attachments. Place the patient in seated position so that gravity plays its normal role. Stand behind the patient and push both thumbs behind the pubic symphysis and then inferiorly *(Illustration 3-29)*. Pushing in different directions provides important information. Pain occurring when you push your fingers against the posterior part of the iliopubic rami results from anteversion. Pain when you push your fingers from the symphysis toward the coccyx results from retroversion. Pain when you push your fingers from one iliopubic ramus toward the opposite sacroiliac joint results from uterine sidebending.

Carefully question the patient to confirm that the pain caused by this test is of the same type and in the same place as the pain she usually experiences. Pushing in the opposite direction should immediately relieve the pain; often, the patient already knows this. Simple coughing or sneezing may aggravate the pain and reveal the zone of adhesion. Lifting of the small intestine and greater omentum can considerably diminish pain caused by abnormal uterine positioning. This underlines the important role of the intestine and abdominal cavitary pressures.

## VAGINAL ROUTE

Place the patient in supine position with bent legs slightly apart. Should the practitioner use a glove during vaginal exams? The bare finger may be more sensitive for detecting hormonal impregnation of the cervix, alteration in texture, and presence of Nabothian follicles. On the other hand, a glove protects both patient and practitioner from the non-negligible risks of infection. In our opinion, a glove does not seriously hinder testing or manipulation, and should therefore be used routinely. Practitioners should try different types of gloves to see which works the best for them.

### Anterior Structures

Place the pad of the finger against the anterior vaginal wall. The vesicovaginal septum is 6-8mm thick here.

URETHRAL SEGMENT: Inferiorly, you can test for a possible urethrocele or fibrosis of the pubo-urethral ligaments (Illustration 3-30). If there is a fibrosis, the urethra resists being stretched upward against the pubis.

BLADDER NECK/TRIGONE: The finger meets these structures on a horizontal going through the inferior part of the pubis, 2-3cm posteriorly. With inflammation of this region or vesicocervical ptosis, the finger detects a protuberance which compresses the anterior vaginal wall. Normally, the bladder neck/trigonal region is felt as a discrete unit. With injury, mobilization of this region provokes pain, an urge to urinate, or (in severe cases) actual urination. Dyspareunia in the prone position with incomplete penetration may also be associated with injuries to this region.

With your finger facing the bladder neck/trigonal region, ask the patient to push down with effort. Normally, the bladder neck should move slightly posteroinferiorly (Illustration 3-31).

With an anterior restriction, the bladder neck will not move. With a posterior restriction, it does move (it is already in a posteroinferior position) but does not come back during a retention effort. With a tear, the movement is ample but painful.

### Posterior Structures

Your finger will detect the perineal and rectal regions via the posterior vaginal wall. The rectouterine pouch may be sensitive when fibrous or invaded by a loop of the

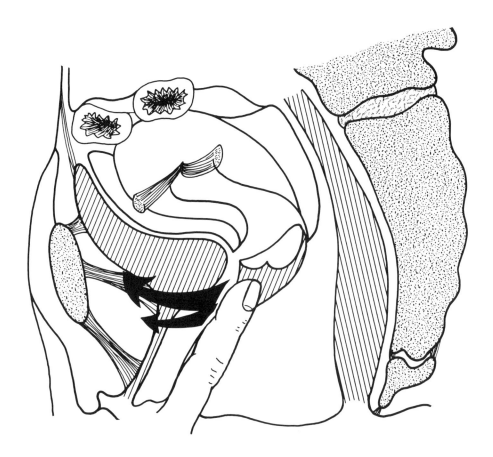

**Illustration 3-30**
Urethral Segment Test

small intestine or an elytrocele. The existence of the pouch (located about 6cm from the anus) should be verified by rectovaginal exam.

## Lateral Structures

Certain pelvic subperitoneal tissues can be tested. The vagina is too easily distended to give much information. It is better to test the cervix/isthmus region.

ELEVATOR FASCICULI OF LEVATOR ANI: With the fingers just above the vulval orifice, at the most anterior part of the pelvic floor, ask the patient to carry out a retention effort *(Illustration 3-32)*. This consists of an isometric contraction opposed by the adductors. During the retention effort, you should feel a cord stretch. Weak tension of this cord reflects hypotonia of the elevator fasciculi.

FASCICULI OF SPHINCTERS: To test tonicity of these fasciculi, move the two intra-vaginal fingers laterally in the direction of the pelvic cavity, and ask the patient to contract the sphincters as if resisting the urge to urinate. This test will enable you to distinguish normal tonicity from hypotonicity or hypertonicity.

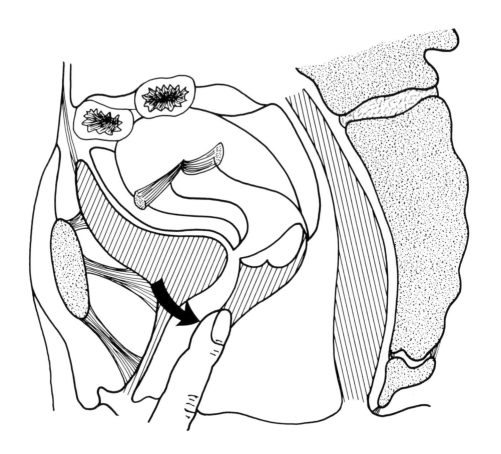

**Illustration 3-31**
Bladder Neck Test with Effort

## Superior Structures

CERVIX: The intravaginal segment which protrudes into the vagina is also known as Tench's snout. The late nineteenth-century anatomist Dubois noted that it has the same consistency and sensation as the nasal alae (Testut, 1889) Two lateral pouches exist in addition to both the anterior and posterior pouches. The uterine body is normally found in the anterior pouch, aside from cases of verticalization or retroversion. The vaginal exam can reveal cases of cervicitis with increased volume of the cervix, edema, and sometimes sclerosis, often presenting the "pepper grain" texture of Nabothian follicles. The posterior pouch is divided in two by the uterosacral ligaments and parametrium. The superior and inferior portions are, respectively, the rectouterine cavity and the rectouterine pouch.

LENGTHENING OF THE CERVIX: When the suspensory structures of the cervix are released, it no longer presses against the anococcygeal body during effort. If the vaginal

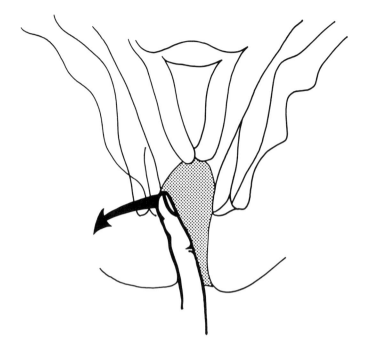

**Illustration 3-32**
Levator Ani Test

fornices remain in good condition, we are likely to see hypertrophic lengthening of the intravaginal part of the cervix. The pouches get deeper and the cervix continues to move downward. The anterior labium of the cervix tends to lengthen more than the posterior labium. With a prolapse, the pouches progressively disappear.

While the uterine body is mobile, the cervix is relatively fixed because of its vaginal insertion, which is, in turn, stabilized by the levators and base of the parametrium, condensed into several folds in the supravaginal portion: i.e., uterosacral, pubovesical, and uterovesical ligaments, and base of the broad ligaments.

UTEROSACRAL LIGAMENTS: Push the posterior part of the cervix anterolaterally *(Illustration 3-33).* Pain indicates abnormal ligamentous tension, or a tear of either the uterosacrals or posterior layers of the broad ligaments.

Observe whether the cervix returns easily to its original position after the mobilization. If it shows little anterior movement and has difficulty returning to its original position, there is a restriction with adhesion of the uterosacrals and posterior part of the broad ligaments. If the cervix shows a sidebending rotation, there is an ipsilateral restriction or a contralateral tear. If the cervix moves too easily and returns to its original position with great difficulty, there is bilateral distention or tear.

PUBOVESICAL AND UTEROVESICAL LIGAMENTS: If these ligaments are fibrosed, the cervix will be anteflexed. If they are lax or torn, the cervix will be retroflexed by the tension of the uterosacral ligaments. Push the anterior part of the cervix posteriorly

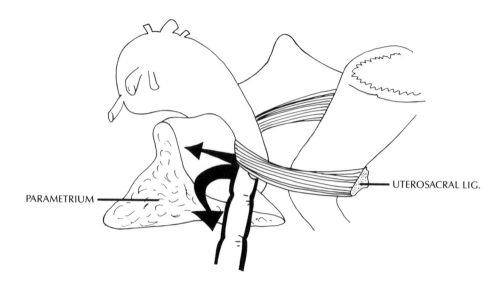

PARAMETRIUM

UTEROSACRAL LIG.

**Illustration 3-33**
Uterosacral Ligament Test

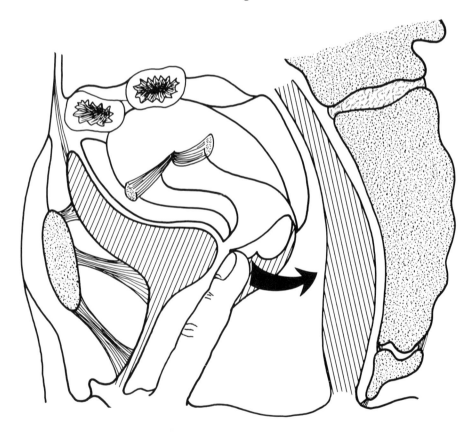

**Illustration 3-34**
Pubovesical and Uterovesical Ligament Test

*(Illustration 3-34)*. If the cervix moves little, and returns to its original position with difficulty, these ligaments are fibrosed. This type of problem is almost always bilateral.

If the cervix is excessively mobile, and does not return to its original position, the anterior ligaments are distended. This is rare.

## Ptoses and Prolapses

With a ptosis, the uterine body and cervix/isthmus region move inferiorly in the pelvic cavity and lose their normal contiguous relationships with adjacent organs. The cervix moves below the transverse plane passing through the sacrococcygeal joint.

With a prolapse, the cervix/isthmus region moves into the vagina. There are three degrees of prolapse, as described earlier. A combination of ptosis and prolapse is the most severe condition.

## Pushing and Retention Tests

The tests discussed so far in this section are passive. They provide information about the distensibility of attachment structures, not their contractility. We have already described pushing tests for the bladder neck/trigonal region. The protocol is the same for the cervix. With pushing efforts, place your fingers in the posterior pouch to evaluate the movement and contraction of the structures around your fingers.

The vaginal dome and cervix form a single organ, held up by the arch of the parametrium and uterosacral ligaments. With release of the posterior suspensory system, the cervix tends to collapse posteriorly with abdominal pushing. With a retention effort, elevation of the cervix is weak or non-existent. To test the suspensory structures, place your fingers in the anterior pouch and have the patient make a retention effort.

## Abdominovaginal Test

For greater clarity, we have been describing the vaginal tests as if they were isolated. In actual practice, they are usually performed as part of a bimanual technique, which makes them complete and precise. For this abdominovaginal test, the abdominal hand palpates the fundus, starting out 3cm above the pubic symphysis and then moving posteroinferiorly. The vaginal and abdominal fingers move toward each other, and evaluate the intervening tissues *(Illustration 3-35)*.

## RECTAL ROUTE

For reasons explained in chapter 2, we prefer to perform the rectal exam with the patient in prone position, legs spread slightly. Place the pad of your index finger against the sacrococcygeal joint and test the rectouterine pouch, cervix, and coccyx *(Illustration 3-36)*. Check for the possible presence of hemorrhoids, which can irritate a posterior uterine restriction.

## Rectouterine Pouch

Test this pouch by pushing on the anterior rectal wall, approximately 6cm from the anus. Evaluate its elasticity. Painful mobilization can result from uterine retroversion,

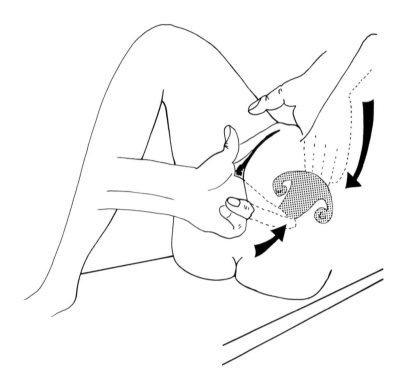

**Illustration 3-35**
Abdominovaginal Test

scarring, or infection. Extreme pain can signify acute infection, severe endometriosis, or tumor. In this situation, gently treat the tissues around the hypersensitive zone in order to release contractures. If the pain persists, send the patient to a specialist for examination and imaging studies.

## Cervix

If you can feel the mass of the cervix when pressing the anterior rectal wall, the cervix is retroposed. To test it, push it forward. If the uterosacral ligaments are fixed, the cervix will be brought slightly anterior and pain will be provoked. If only one uterosacral ligament is fixed, the cervix will move forward and bend toward the injured side.

First, determine whether the uterine body is perceptible in the anterior pouch. Next, explore the parametrium, broad ligaments, uterine tubes, and ovaries. Your hands should very delicately cause the tissues to slide upon each other, following vertical and horizontal directions. If you encounter a guarding reaction or contracture, find out its origin. Be extremely cautious and gentle in manipulating the ovaries. If you have any reason to suspect a tumor, acute infection, etc., send the patient to an appropriate specialist.

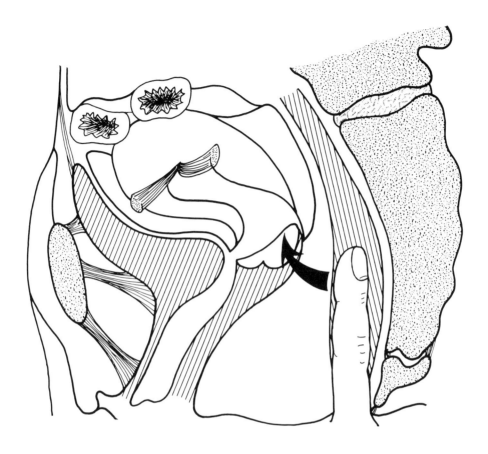

**Illustration 3-36**
Rectal Exam

## Rectovaginal Exam

This exam was described in chapter 2. It allows you to evaluate the thickness and consistency of the perineal body, to evaluate the rectovaginal septum, and to check for a possible elytrocele. The latter, during pushing or retention effort by the patient, gives the impression of a granular structure which has a crackling sensation under your fingers.

Try lifting the intestinal/omental mass with your abdominal hand to find out if the small intestine leaves the rectouterine pouch easily. The patient can be taught this technique. This phenomenon is observed mostly in asthenic, depressed, or exhausted individuals.

## Sacrococcygeal Joint

It is preferable to evaluate sacrococcygeal problems with one finger in the rectum, pressing on the internal surface of the coccyx, and the thumb pressing on the external surface *(Illustration 3-37)*. If compression provokes pain within the coccyx, this usually

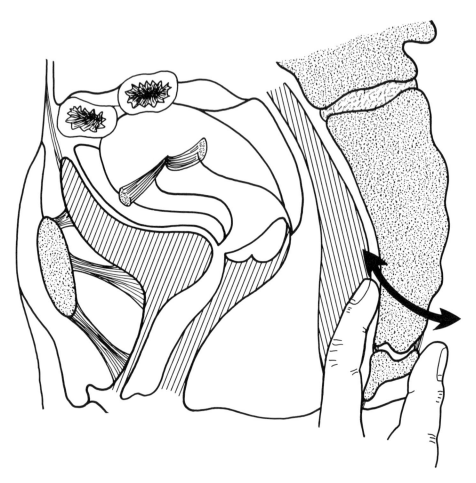

**Illustration 3-37**
Sacrococcygeal Test: Rectal Route

indicates an articular restriction. If pain is felt outside the coccyx, the restriction is more likely to be perineal or parametrial.

An anterior flexion lesion of the coccyx can result from restrictions to the perineum or parametrium that stretch the anococcygeal body and pull the perineal body posteriorly. A purely sacrococcygeal restriction is more likely to relax the anococcygeal body.

## Positioning

A guarding position is more commonly observed in association with stress incontinence than with uterine restrictions. However, in the latter case you may still see external rotation and adduction of the legs, anterior pubic projection, and contraction of the gluteals. These actions represent attempts to increase the efficiency of the internal and external obturators, pyramidalis, levator ani, and sphincter muscles.

When the irritation is near the ovaries and lateral aspect of the broad ligaments, the patient tends to keep her legs in external rotation and the spine kyphosed. This position is due to the psoas and the iliac fascia, which are traversed by the iliohypogastric, ilioinguinal, femoral cutaneous, genitofemoral, obturator, and femoral nerves. The subperitoneal iliolumbar connective tissue communicates with the connective tissue of the broad ligaments, which leads to interdependence between the psoas and pelvis. Typically, the patient will prefer to lift the stomach to release abdominal pressure, raise the legs to improve disturbed pelvic circulation, and lie in the prone position.

## *Motility Test*

The motility of the uterus is similar to that of the bladder, probably because of their common embryological origin. Place the palm of one hand on the suprapubic region, and the other hand under the sacrum. The patient should be in supine or lateral decubitus position (the latter to prevent the sacral hand from being crushed by the weight of the pelvis). During inspir, the abdominal hand moves anteroinferiorly, while the sacral hand moves posterosuperiorly *(Illustration 3-38)*.

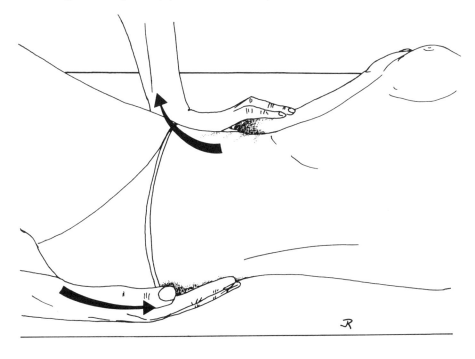

**Illustration 3-38**
Motility Test: Inspir

When there is a restriction, movement takes place in a frontal or transverse rather than sagittal plane, depending upon the location of the problem. Without exception, the hand is drawn toward the restriction, which then becomes the new axis of movement.

We have carried out many experiments on fibroses, ovarian cysts, myomas, endometriosis, etc., described on paper the specific area to which our hand was drawn, and compared these results with ultrasound and radiological evaluations. With very few exceptions, our localizations were exactly correct.

## General Listening

The patient should sit in a kyphosed position, legs slightly apart. Stand behind her, one hand on the skull, the other under the sacrum. The body will always sidebend to the side of the restriction. The greater the degree of sidebending, the further down in the body is the restriction (see *Illustration 1-2* on page 10, and corresponding text).

In general, the only part of the uterus that can be "heard" in general listening is the cervix. With posterior restrictions of the uterosacral ligaments, the head goes very far back and down. When only one side is affected, there is sidebending toward that side. These motions are very similar to those resulting from coccygeal restrictions. The only way to distinguish them is to slightly compress the skull (push it inferiorly) prior to general listening. If general listening is unchanged or the motion is more obvious, the problem is probably sacrococcygeal; if the motion is less obvious, the problem is probably in the urogenital system.

With anterior restrictions of the cervix, the head bends far down toward the pubic symphysis. With restriction of an ovary, the motion is similar but with the addition of sidebending toward the affected ovary. This motion is so characteristic of pelvic restrictions that you should always check the pelvis carefully whenever you feel it on general listening.

## Restrictions

Restrictions of the uterus can occur in many directions. Their principal causes are described below.

### Superior

Superior restrictions result either from ptosis or from adhesion of the small intestine, omentum, or peritoneum, all of which are common sequelae of infection or abdominal surgery. These superior structures press against the uterine fundus and disturb the distribution of intracavitary pressures. Diaphragmatic attraction is poorly transmitted and the phenomena of reciprocal tension, turgor effect, and the propulsive and aspirational forces of the cardiovascular system are disturbed. The effective weight of the uterus is increased and it tends to move downward.

### Anterior

Anterior restrictions of the uterus follow retractions of the vesical attachments resulting from inflammation or surgery of the bladder or supravesical tissues. Fixation of the uterovesical pouch can bring the uterus into anteversion or anteflexion. Injury to the vesicovaginal septum and fascia leads to a type of dyspareunia which we have already described. Less commonly, uterine anteversion is due to rupture of the two uterosacral ligaments and the posteroinferior layers of the broad ligaments. This situation does not represent a true restriction because the position of the uterus is easily reducible.

An anterior restriction of the coccyx slackens the tonus of the pelvic floor in a positional or reflex manner:

- positional: the coccyx moves nearer to the pelvic floor, and muscular/aponeurotic fibers are relaxed;
- reflex: the osteoarticular restriction interferes with nervous stimulation and diminishes local tonus. It is very rare for a reflexogenic effect to cause hypertonia.

### Lateral, Posterior

Lateral restrictions of the uterus result from inflammatory, surgical, or obstetrical injuries to the broad ligaments or suspensory ligaments of the ovaries. If only one broad ligament is affected, the uterus will be pulled into sidebending. If both are affected, the uterus is pulled more posteriorly. Restriction of a single uterosacral ligament will also pull the uterus into sidebending.

Posterior restriction usually results from tearing of the uterosacral ligaments during pregnancy or childbirth. During healing of the ligaments, the cervix/isthmus region is drawn posteriorly, and the sacrum is fixed anteriorly.

### Inferior

Inferior restrictions result from pregnancy and childbirth, or (less commonly) from infection or trauma to the coccyx. An injury to the sacrogenital folds, uterosacral ligaments, or perineum can lead to fibrosis of this group of structures, which no longer function effectively as shock-absorbers and distributors of pressures. The uterus is inevitably drawn downward by gravity and pressure from above. If the pelvic floor is hypotonic and slack, the uterus and other pelvic organs will tend to prolapse and migrate toward their orifices.

## *Manipulations*

### CONTRAINDICATIONS

Contraindications to manipulation of the uterus are similar to those described in chapters 1 and 2. We are usually talking about contraindications to direct, internal manipulation. When external manipulations or induction are to be avoided, this will be specifically stated.

### Pregnancy

There are several reliable biochemical tests for pregnancy. Even in this modern age, some patients come to us for internal manipulations unaware that they are pregnant. Some early physical signs of pregnancy are:

- softening of the cervix (it will have the consistency of the tongue);
- increased volume of the uterine body;
- softening of the uterine body (it will have the consistency of a ripe fig).

## Intrauterine Devices

The presence of an intrauterine device (I.U.D.) carries a certain risk of injury or bleeding of the uterine mucosa during direct manipulation. Do not hesitate to have them removed. Inflammation and scarring can lead to restrictions which affect the uterine tubes. Motility techniques may be affected by intrauterine devices if the axis of movement becomes focused on the device. In our experience, only about 20% of intrauterine devices have no influence whatsoever on mobility or motility.

## Ectopic Pregnancy

Manipulation of a patient with an ectopic pregnancy (see chapter 4) can lead to serious hemorrhaging. We have dealt with several women who have consulted us about acute lower back pain when they actually had ectopic pregnancies. This condition presents very few initial symptoms, so you must be very observant and wary. "Red flags" include abnormal paleness, lower back pain with anterior radiation, painful abdomen, intense sensitivity of the para-uterine area, hyperventilation, diminished blood pressure with a thready and rapid pulse, and a missed period. If you encounter some combination of these signs, send the patient to the nearest hospital. Ectopic pregnancies can be life-threatening, and there is no point in taking chances.

## Tumors and Radiation Treatment

Cervical cancer is a definite contraindication to manipulation. This should be evaluated by pap smear, but can sometimes also be felt. The cervix may feel hardened, infiltrated, and irregular. Induration is limited and nodular. Traces of blood may be seen on the glove.

Manipulation of a uterus carrying a tumor can lead to hemorrhage, infection, or even tumor growth or metastasis. If you have reason to suspect cancer (e.g., cervical changes as above, bleeding outside the menstrual period, foul-smelling discharge, local-ized pain, unexplained fever, or unexplained weight-loss), send the patient to a specialist immediately.

Be very careful with women who have had radiation treatment of the pelvis. The tissues will be irritated and fragile. Direct manipulation poses a risk of hemorrhage and tissue injury.

## EXTERNAL MANIPULATIONS

To obtain satisfactory results in treatment of the uterus, it is essential that you test and manipulate (if necessary) the small intestine, greater omentum, median and medial umbilical ligaments, and pubovesical ligaments. Appropriate techniques are described in chapter 2.

## Uterine Body

SUPINE POSITION: The patient lies with hips flexed and feet resting on a small cushion. It is important to manipulate the fundus because it tends to adhere to the peritoneum, and peritoneal restrictions can fix the uterine fundus. Place your fingers about three finger-widths above the pubic symphysis and gently push them into the abdomen, posteriorly, slightly inferiorly, and then posteriorly again. Move the loops of the small intestine out of the way, toward the front or side. When you find the restriction, stretch the tissues anteriorly, inferiorly, and laterally *(Illustration 3-39)*. Begin at the periphery of the restriction and gradually move toward the center. Repeat this until the pain is diminished and the tissues become more supple. This is a fairly difficult process. Three or four treatment sessions are usually required to obtain good results.

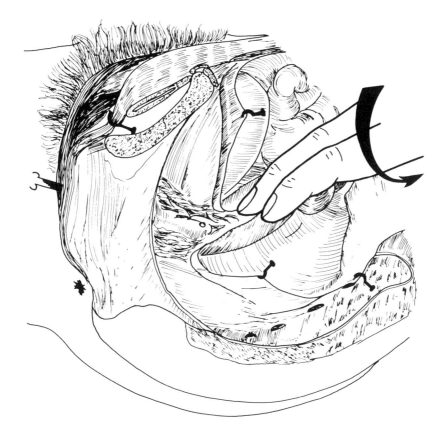

**Illustration 3-39**
Manipulation of Uterine Body: Supine Position

LATERAL DECUBITUS POSITION: The patient lies on one side with hips flexed. Your hands work on the side which is near the table. This is the ideal position for approaching the lateral parts of the uterus. Push the fingers toward the table and pedad under the anterosuperior iliac spines, and then return posteriorly and medially *(Illustration 3-40)*. If you find an area of restriction of the broad ligaments and uterine body, stretch the tissues alternately toward the median axis of the body and then toward the walls of the pelvic cavity. Repeat this rhythmically until you feel a release. The lateral parts of the uterus demand great caution because of the presence of the ovaries: the closer one gets to the ovaries, the gentler and lighter the maneuvers should become.

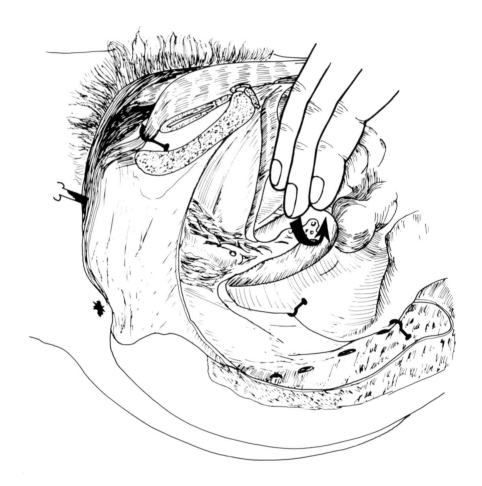

**Illustration 3-40**
Manipulation of Uterine Body: Lateral Decubitus Position

To increase the depth of manipulation, apply one hand to the uterus while using the other to flex the legs. Alternatively, you can fix the restriction under your fingers and indirectly stretch the tissues by mobilizing the legs.

SEATED POSITION: The patient sits in kyphosed position with hands clasped behind the neck and legs slightly apart. To work on the left side, take both the patient's elbows in your right hand and with your left hand treat the deep pelvic region, moving from the iliac arch to the median axis. Retain the flexion and stretch the tissues by passively mobilizing the body (*Illustration 3-41*). This is a good technique for the base and the superolateral parts of the uterus.

KNEE/ELBOW POSITION: In this position, the omentum and small intestine move away from the pelvis and the abdominal musculature is relaxed. Approach the uterus laterally— it will be anteverted and therefore more accessible. Hold the restriction and stretch it by making the pelvis move over the femoral heads. For example, if you find a utero-

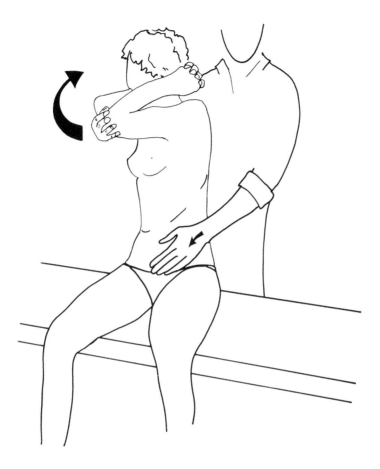

**Illustration 3-41**
Manipulation of Uterine Body: Seated Position

vesical restriction on the uterine body, place your fingers immediately above it to hold it and, with the other hand, push the sacrum anterosuperiorly *(Illustration 3-42)*. This stretches the tissue fibers, as we have verified using fluoroscopy. Repeat this technique over 3-4 sessions for optimal results. Do not perform this technique in the presence of an I.U.D.

MODIFIED TRENDELENBURG POSITION: This position allows you to reach the deeper pelvic tissues. Pull the patient's legs toward her chest, or place one foot on the opposite knee. Starting from the medial edge of the iliac fossa, move your fingers inferomedially toward the uterine axis. If you are working directly on the restricted area, hold it with one hand and use the other hand to move the legs for indirect stretching *(Illustration 3-43)*.

## Sacral Pumping

The uterosacral ligaments and sacrogenital folds originate from S2-S4 and run to the cervix/isthmus part of the uterus or sometimes farther on to the pubis. By the rectal

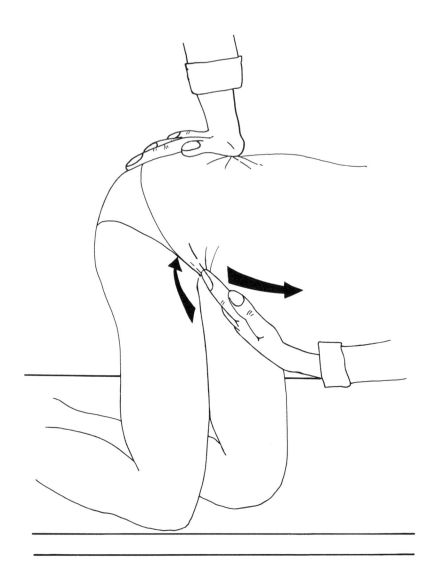

**Illustration 3-42**
Manipulation of Uterine Body: Knee/Elbow Position

route, you can reach the anterolateral parts of these structures. However, when their posterior attachments are restricted the anterior sacrum is blocked. These restrictions can be released by "pumping" the sacrum. Place the patient in prone position, a cushion under the pelvis. Using both hands, rhythmically push the sacrum as follows *(Illustration 3-44)*:

- anteroinferiorly to put pressure on S1-S2;
- straight anteriorly to put pressure on S2-S3;
- anterosuperiorly to put pressure on S4-C1.

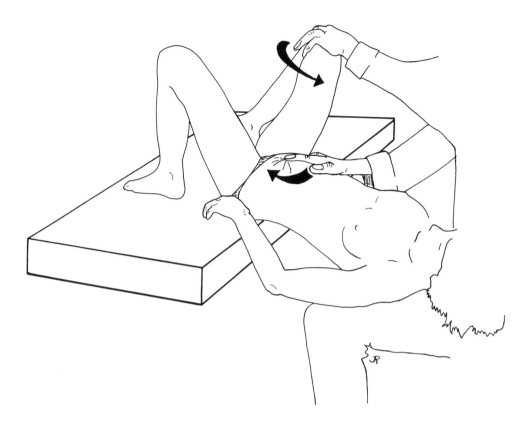

**Illustration 3-43**
Manipulation of Uterine Body: Modified Trendelenburg Position

The movements should be well separated in order to increase their efficacy. The sacrum is often fixed anteriorly. To relax the ligaments, push the sacrum anteriorly to return it to its original position. Doing this repeatedly and rhythmically brings the anterior structures into play and facilitates their release. This is a compression technique, in which the tissues are released by moving into the restriction.

With a lateral injury, the sacrum tends to move anteriorly by rotation on the contralateral side. Do not try to correct the blocked zone, but go into the restriction and mobilize the sacrum on its mobile side. After several rotation movements, the retracted fibers will gradually relax and the sacrum will resume its normal anteroposterior movement.

Sacral pumping enlivens the tissues and makes them more dynamic. In part this is done via the innervation of the sacral plexus. Always check sacral mechanics after this technique and treat any remaining restrictions.

## Sacrococcygeal Pumping

This technique is used when, in addition to uterosacral restriction, the anococcygeal body is overstretched. It demonstrates participation of the pericoccygeal fibers in

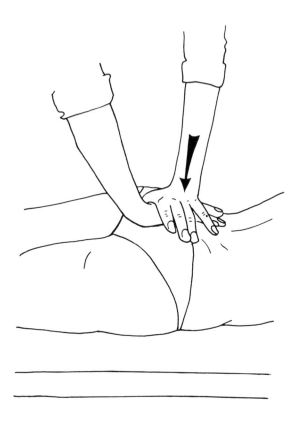

**Illustration 3-44**
Sacral Pumping

sacral restriction. With the patient in prone position, place your hand and arm along the longitudinal axis of the sacrum. Press the heel of your hand on the coccyx and your fingers on the sacrum. Push the coccyx inferiorly, slightly anteriorly, then superiorly, and let it return. Repeat the technique in synchrony with the tissues' natural rhythm.

## Obturator Foramen

Treatment of this region was discussed in chapter 2. The patient lies supine, with legs apart. The leg on the treated side is bent and the other leg straight. Place your hand under the anterior adductors, thumb under pectineus and adductor magnus, index finger on gracilis. Slide your fingers around the adductors until you are in contact with the external obturator, obturator membrane, and internal obturator. Wiggle your thumb slightly until it is as close as possible to the obturator foramen, and stretch the tissues *(Illustration 3-45)*.

This stimulatory technique increases intra-obturator pressure and triggers a reflex effect to change the height of the bladder and uterus (confirmed using fluoroscopy) and contract the perineum. This involves the obturator muscles, obturator membrane, and its attachments which are shared with the levator ani. Carry out movements of the hip

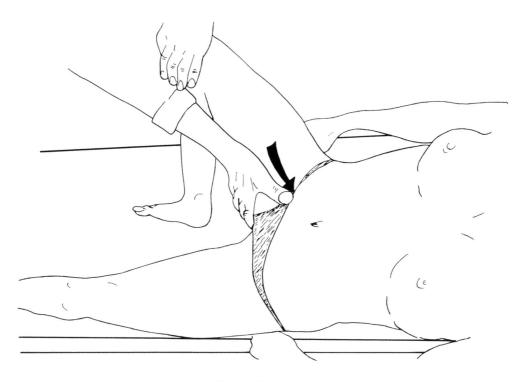

**Illustration 3-45**
Manipulation of Obturator Foramen

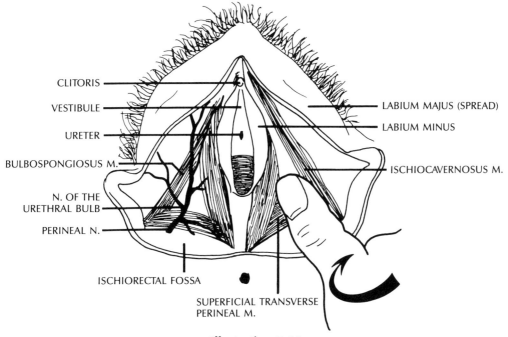

CLITORIS

VESTIBULE

URETER

BULBOSPONGIOSUS M.

N. OF THE
URETHRAL BULB

PERINEAL N.

LABIUM MAJUS (SPREAD)

LABIUM MINUS

ISCHIOCAVERNOSUS M.

ISCHIORECTAL FOSSA

SUPERFICIAL TRANSVERSE
PERINEAL M.

**Illustration 3-46**
Manipulation of Anterior Perineum

joint and move your thumb in deeper during each internal rotation and adduction. During this process, your other fingers can work on the ischiorectal region (discussed below).

This technique is designed to stretch peri- and intra-obturator adhesions when they are accessible and, via a reflex route, to increase the tone of the contractile fibers. When the thumb is in place, you can utilize diaphragmatic respiration (intrapelvic pressure is typically highest at the end of exhalation). Occasionally (because of obesity, tension, etc.) you will not be able to reach the obturator foramen with your thumb. In this case, go as far as possible between the iliac and ischial pubic rami in order to press against the insertions.

### Anterior Perineum

This is the pre-ischiatic part of the perineal body. Place one or two fingers or the thumb on either side of the anterior commissure of the vulva and labia majora (which should remain closed). Push posterolaterally to stretch fibrosed regions on the ischiopubic rami (Illustration 3-46). Then move your fingers from the ischiopubic ramus toward the pubis, pressing on the superficial perineal aponeurosis, urogenital diaphragm, bulbospongiosus, ischiocavernosus, and superficial transversalis. This is a technique that should always be performed on women who have had an episiotomy.

OBTURATOR NERVE: This is found three finger-widths lateral to the pubic symphysis, along the iliopubic ramus. Perineal structures are stimulated by pressing gently 2 or 3 times on this area.

### Ischiorectal Fossa

SUPINE POSITION: Your hand stretches the ischiorectal region, moving from the medial edge of the ischium toward the perineal body and anus, and then back. For an indirect technique, hold the fixed zone with one hand and stretch the tissues via the flexors and abductors of the leg.

SEATED POSITION: Position the patient as for the coccyx test. While pressure is on one ischium, place your fingers under the restriction, then return the patient to normal bi-ischiatic pressure. All inter-ischial structures will already be separated. Press the fixed fibers superolaterally (Illustration 3-47). You can also mobilize the body by rotating the torso on the pelvis (patient's hands clasped behind her neck), in order to bring one ischium anterolaterally. With practice, you will be able to place the other hand on the ischium to increase the amplitude of the movements.

### Stretching via Leg Muscles

Para-uterine restrictions can be treated and released via polyarticular leg muscles and associated membranes. Our work has clearly shown that stretching or contraction of specific leg muscles affects specific pelvic organs or connective structures. Some of these techniques can be practiced by the patient at home, with appropriate instruction. They can prolong and increase the benefits of your manipulation by preventing the tissues from retracting again afterwards.

ADDUCTION AND INTERNAL ROTATION: The internal and external obturator muscles, pyramidalis, and quadratus femoris are primarily abductors and external rotators.

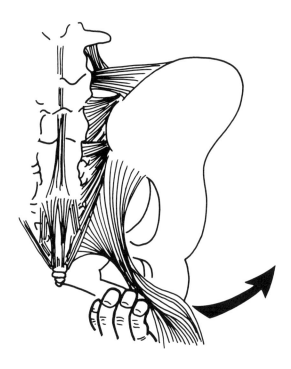

**Illustration 3-47**
Manipulation of Ischiorectal Fossa

They have many direct and indirect connections with urogenital structures, and stretching these muscles can release intrapelvic microadhesions. With the patient in supine position, place the treated leg on top of the other and use your hand to adduct and internally rotate it *(Illustration 3-48)*. You should always determine beforehand if limitation of hip rotation is due to some osteoarticular factor. With joint problems, mobilization produces acute pain in the fold of the groin, which is greatly increased by intra-articular compression. This type of compressive pain is not observed with secondary retractions of the pelvitrochanteric muscles.

SACROSPINOUS AND SACROTUBEROUS LIGAMENTS: These ligaments insert on the sacrum, coccyx, sciatic spine, and ischium. Because of their relationships with the coccygeus, levator ani, internal obturator, and their aponeuroses, stretching of these ligaments affects the uterus and other intrapelvic organs. The patient is supine with one leg bent. Bring the bent leg into flexion, adduction, and internal rotation (the other leg remains flat on the table), in order to move the ischium away from the sacral axis. You can also accomplish this with the patient in seated position by moving one knee toward the opposite shoulder.

BICEPS FEMORIS: The distal insertion of the biceps femoris is on the head of the fibula (a well-known reflex zone), and its proximal origin shares fibers with the sacrotuberous ligament. It is therefore interesting to accompany stretching of the sacrospinous and sacrotuberous ligaments with that of the biceps femoris. The patient sits with both legs

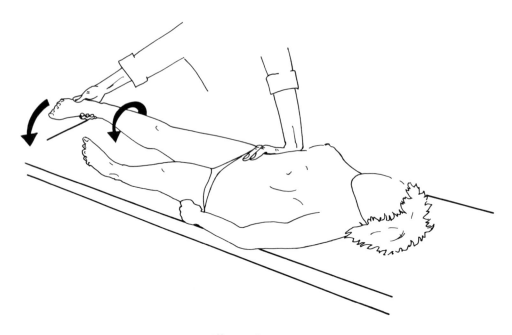

**Illustration 3-48**
Stretching of Internal Obturator

stretched out, her torso is pushed toward the non-treated side, and her leg on the treated side is internally rotated *(Illustration 3-49)*. You can teach the patient to do this at home.

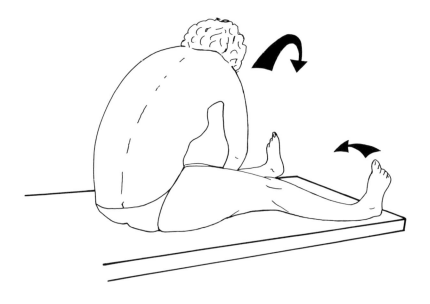

**Illustration 3-49**
Stretching of Biceps Femoris

ROUND LIGAMENTS: These ligaments have numerous tiny connections with the inguinal canal and inguinal ligament. They can be defibrosed by placing the patient in supine position and extending and adducting the leg on the treated side. This technique should be performed routinely on a uterus which is anteverted or generally restricted.

TONIFICATION: Besides stretching as described above, the fibers of the pelvitrochanteric muscles can be tonified by isometric contraction. Teach your patients to do these isometric exercises at home. Homework should include the well-known pelvic tonification techniques (retention exercises during deep breathing and coughing).

We also ask patients to mentally "tune in" to the tensions they feel in the pelvis in both the standing and knee-elbow positions. They can then focus, release areas of excess tension, and balance the tensions. These techniques are not as difficult as they sound, and most women enjoy doing them.

## ABDOMINOVAGINAL ROUTE

The bimanual exam permits very precise release of tissue restrictions. When a zone of restriction is localized, the vaginal and abdominal fingers move to meet each other while separating out the different tissues they meet. Different fibrous or muscular layers are freed by sliding upon each other, like two sheets of paper.

Abdominovaginal manipulation is most appropriate for problems of the uterine pouches. Specific techniques depend upon the position of the uterus (anteversion or retroversion) and cervix (anteposition or retroposition). Experience has shown us that it is the position of the cervix that is most important. *Our techniques are not intended to put the uterus and cervix back into position, but to restore their mobility.* With this understanding we avoid therapeutic relentlessness and potential disillusionment.

You can put one or two intravaginal fingers into the uterine pouches, depending upon their shape, but we will refer to one finger for the sake of simplicity. These techniques can be performed in the prone, supine, or lateral decubitus positions, depending upon the status of the cervix. Each of these techniques should be repeated four or five times, rhythmically, for best results.

Local listening can be combined with any of the following techniques. It is especially helpful for the intravaginal hand. With your hand in place, do local listening and then allow your fingers to go in the direction of the motion they feel. Doing this, while keeping in mind the importance of gentle and rhythmic movements, will often lead to significant releases.

### Possible Combinations of Uterine Anteversion/Retroversion and Cervical Anteposition/Retroposition

ANTEVERSION/ANTEPOSITION: The patient is in supine position. Your abdominal hand searches for the uterine fundus under the superior part of the symphysis. Your intravaginal finger is in the anterior pouch (which is only barely palpable in this case), or on the superior part of the anterior vaginal wall. The hands carry out 4 or 5 posteroinferior movements, followed by 2 or 3 superior movements *(Illustration 3-50)*.

ANTEVERSION/RETROPOSITION: The patient is in lateral decubitus position. Your abdominal hand performs the same movement as in the technique above. Your intravaginal finger is in the rectouterine pouch or on the superior part of the posterior vaginal wall. The two hands go toward each other and move superiorly *(Illustration 3-51)*.

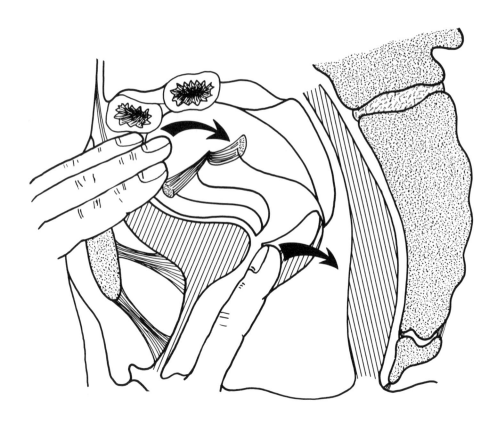

**Illustration 3-50**
Uterine Anteversion/ Cervical Anteposition

RETROVERSION/ANTEPOSITION:  The patient is supine. Your intravaginal finger is in the anterior vaginal pouch or on the superior part of the anterior vaginal wall. Push this finger posteriorly while the abdominal fingers laterally approach the uterine body and pull it anteriorly *(Illustration 3-52)*.

RETROVERSION/RETROPOSITION:  The patient is in lateral decubitus position. Your intravaginal finger is in the rectouterine pouch or on the superior part of the posterior vaginal wall, and pushes the cervix anteriorly. The abdominal fingers obliquely approach the lateral aspects of the uterus and push it anteriorly *(Illustration 3-53)*.

## Uterine and Cervical Lateral Deviation

Significant lateral deviation of the uterus and cervix is seldom considered in conventional medical texts. Nevertheless, it does occur and can eventually affect the adnexal system (see chapter 4).

Treatment is relatively simple. For a right lateral deviation, place the patient in left lateral decubitus position (to enlist the aid of gravity). Place your intravaginal finger in the right lateral pouch or corresponding superior part of the vagina. Push the cervix to the left. Simultaneously, place your abdominal hand to the right of the uterus and push it to the left *(Illustration 3-54)*.

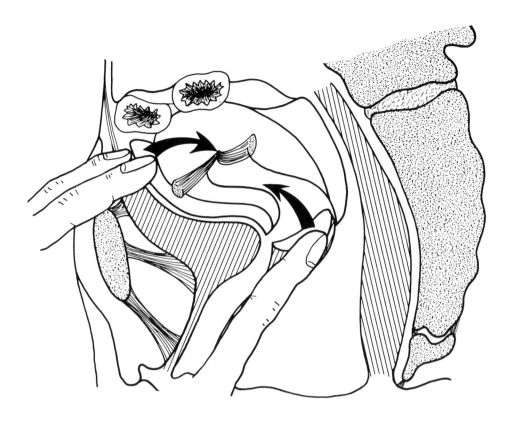

**Illustration 3-51**
Uterine Anteversion/ Cervical Retroposition

Obviously, many combinations and degrees of uterine and cervical restrictions are possible. The greater your experience, the more adept you will become at finding the best position and technique for dealing with individual cases.

## Pushing and Retention Techniques

These techniques can help in mobilization of the cervix. Consider a retroposition. While you manipulate it anterosuperiorly, ask the patient to make a retention effort. This will improve the cervical correction. When you manipulate an anteposition, ask the patient to make a pushing effort. These efforts by the patient will also stimulate the important local muscular fibers.

## Ptoses and Prolapses

None of our manipulative techniques are helpful for third degree prolapses. However, we can deal with ptoses (or even first and second degree prolapses), and alleviate the discomfort and pain which they cause. In several ptosis cases we have treated, radiography has revealed a normalization of interstructural relationships. However, we reiterate that positional reduction *per se* is not our goal. A ptosed uterus or cervix is functional as long as it is mobile.

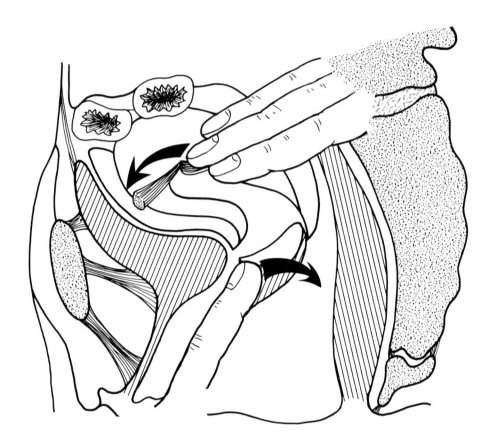

**Illustration 3-52**
Uterine Retroversion/ Cervical Anteposition

To treat a ptosis, have the patient lie prone with pelvis resting on a cushion to protect the anterosuperior iliac spines. Place both intravaginal fingers on the anterior and posterior pouches, on the two lateral pouches, or (if these cannot be found) on the circumference of the cervix. Push superiorly with these fingers, while your abdominal hand approaches the uterine body laterally on the left and then right and pushes it superiorly (Illustration 3-55).

Ultimately, our aim is not to simply manipulate a cervical retroposition or whatever, but to release retractions or restrictions of the uterosacral and broad ligaments and other supporting structures.

## RECTAL ROUTE

### Cervical Retroposition

Retracted and fibrosed uterosacral ligaments can also be freed via the rectal route. Remember that the cervix is at the same level as the sacrococcygeal joint. With the

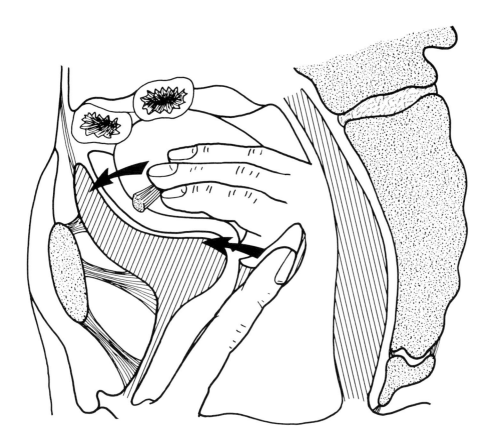

**Illustration 3-53**
Uterine Retroversion/ Cervical Retroposition

patient prone, push the intrarectal finger against the anterior rectal wall, anteriorly and slightly superiorly. You will feel the round mass of the cervix if it is retroposed. Push it rhythmically forward several times. This technique is generally less effective than those described above, but does have the single advantage of freeing the posterior part of the rectouterine pouch.

**Vaginorectal Technique**

This permits the freeing of certain uncommon adhesions of the vaginorectal septum associated with an elytrocele. It can also be used for significant fibroses of the rectouterine pouch (situated 6cm above the anus). Slide the intravaginal and intrarectal fingers against each other as if rubbing two sheets of paper together. Continue doing this, paying close attention to the feel of the tissues, until you feel a release.

**COCCYX**

Coccygeal techniques were described in detail in Chapter 2 (pages 75-79). Coccygeal restrictions in women are common, resulting from childbirth, direct trauma, or other

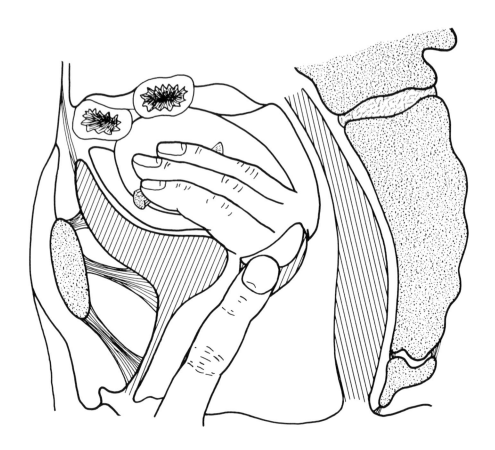

**Illustration 3-54**
Uterine and Cervical Lateral Deviation

causes. Manipulation of the uterus or bladder must always be accompanied by treatment of the coccyx.

## Posterior Restrictions

These are seen almost exclusively in women. During childbirth, the head of the fetus pushes the coccyx posteriorly, sometimes dislocating it. The anterior sacrococcygeal ligament is stretched, whereas the posterior sacrococcygeal ligament gradually shortens, fibroses, and keeps the coccyx in its extended position.

Sometimes, while performing the test in seated position, the mere pressure from your finger will free the coccyx and "put it back into place." We routinely emphasize mobility over position, so this is the only time you will see this phrase in this book. But the phrase is appropriate in this case, since the articular surfaces involved can move by more than 5mm. Adjustment of this positional restriction gives very dramatic positive results.

The seated position is preferable because the pericoccygeal muscles and ligaments create a corrective tension. Place the palm of your hand over the sacrum, fingers on the

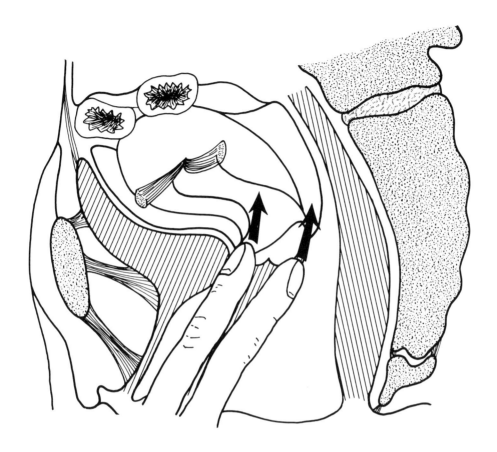

**Illustration 3-55**
Manipulation of Ptosed Uterus

coccyx, and move the coccyx anterosuperiorly *(Illustration 3-56)*. The adjustment may be easier if you use your other hand to slightly compress the skull.

Alternatively, put the patient in supine position, legs slightly apart. Place your pisiform or adjacent part of the hypothenar eminence against the coccyx, take up the slack, and make an anterosuperior adjustment.

Unlike an anterior restriction, a posterior restriction does not directly affect the perineal tissues. However, it does have a reflex effect which leads to spasms and hardening of the perineum. This perineal spasm brings the urogenital system into a chronic retentive position, congests the pelvis, and irritates many sensitive fibers. This gives a more medial pain sensation.

## Anterior Restrictions

These are seen in both women and men, and are typically sequelae of falls and direct traumas. Corrective techniques using the rectal route were described in detail in chapter 2. The prone position is preferable, and proper placement of your intrarectal finger is crucial *(Illustration 3-57)*.

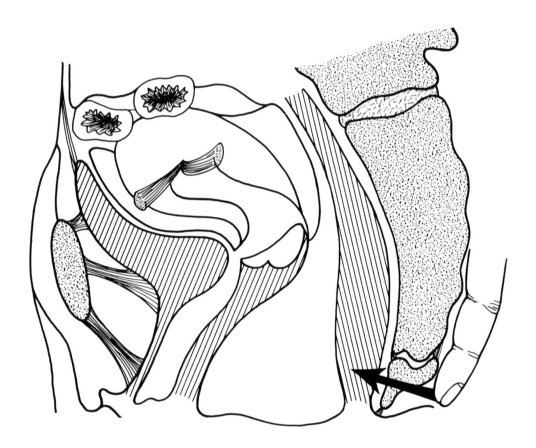

**Illustration 3-56**
Manipulation of Posterior Coccygeal Restriction

An anterior restriction relaxes the perineum, and brings the urogenital system into a chronic pushing position. This leads, progressively, to general ptosis of the viscera. In these cases the pain is experienced primarily posteriorly.

## Tonification Techniques

PERINEUM: Techniques for tonifying the perineum (see chapter 2) help maintain and prolong the effects of manipulation. You should teach the patient to do them at home. Our fluoroscopic studies indicate that the most effective movements are:

- Supine, hips flexed, with a cushion between the legs. Press the knees together and act as if resisting the urge to urinate (retention effort). Repeat about thirty times.
- Supine, legs extended. Push the pubis anteriorly, press the lateral sides of the feet against the floor, and exert retention effort. Also repeat this about thirty times.

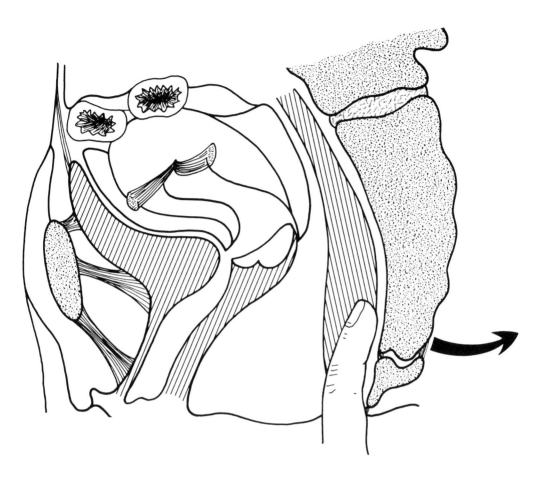

**Illustration 3-57**
Manipulation of Anterior Coccygeal Restriction

SPHINCTERS AND LEVATORS: This technique consists of stopping and starting urination several times in a row. It serves first to make the patient aware of the perineal
region and the sphincters and is also a tonifying exercise. Often, patients no longer have
sufficient local and central stimulation so they should either try during sexual intercourse
to squeeze the penis or to place an object into the vagina and practice with that. This
will help them become aware of the contractions of the levator ani and to reinforce them
by stimulating them several times.

# *Motility*

## UTEROSACRAL INDUCTION

Induction techniques are the same as those for the bladder. With the patient in
lateral decubitus position, place one hand on the abdomen facing the fundus, and the

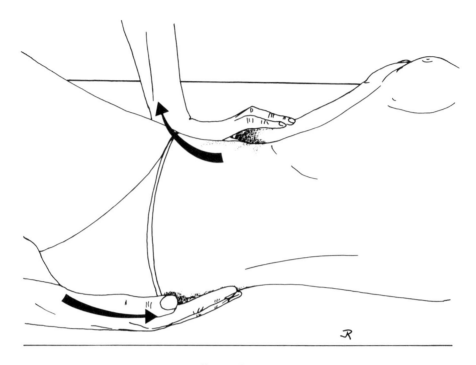

**Illustration 3-58**
Uterosacral Induction

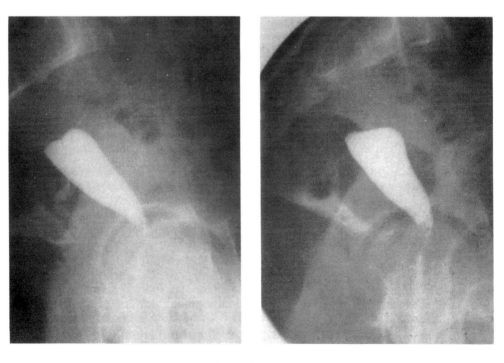

**Illustration 3-59**
Effect of Uterosacral Induction on a Retroverted Uterus

other on the sacrum. In inspir, the urogenital axis moves slightly anteroinferiorly, while the sacrum moves posterosuperiorly. Expir is just the opposite *(Illustration 3-58)*. Induction consists of following the motion and accentuating the phase with greater amplitude, but without inhibiting anything. Remember that the axis of motion is often altered when there are significant pelvic restrictions. Continue this until the motion normalizes, which may occur with or without a release.

### Radiographic Evidence

We have long had the goal of documenting motility (i.e., cyclical subtle motion of visceral organs not caused by the diaphragm), but this has proved extremely difficult to do with sufficient scientific rigor. However, we have been able to use fluoroscopy to demonstrate the effect of uterosacral induction on the slightly retroverted uterus of a female patient with three children. Following the fourth induction movement, the uterus normalized itself by 20-30° *(Illustration 3-59)*. These before-and-after photographs clearly show the change in position, even though the axis of motion is somewhat altered. This is a striking illustration of the power of induction techniques.

## LUMBOGENITAL INDUCTION

We believe that this technique has a significant effect on the suspensory ligaments of the ovaries, although we have not been able to document this conclusively. The patient is supine, with hips flexed. Place one hand under the lower three lumbar vertebrae and the other on the abdomen, over the base of the uterus. The movement is one of frontal sliding—during expir, the abdominal hand moves mostly superiorly while the lumbar hand moves inferiorly *(Illustration 3-60)*. Follow until the motion normalizes.

## GENERAL INDUCTION

With the patient in supine position, place one hand on the restricted area and use your other hand to hold the legs. The abdominal hand induces the injured fibers. With general listening technique, the body always "closes up" around the injured zone, and the legs move into sidebending and rotation on the restricted side. The angle between the restriction and the legs becomes more and more acute. Then a breakthrough point is reached where the angle becomes less acute, and the injured fibers become slightly stretched and defibrosed, gradually regaining their normal distensibility. During this time, the abdominal hand finds and restrains the tightest zones, which must then be released specifically. We find this technique especially helpful in complex cases, e.g., when the small intestine, bladder, and uterus are all involved.

The treatment sequence during a typical session in the presence of a significant restriction is as follows:

- mobility and motility tests;
- direction manipulation;
- local induction;
- general induction;
- local induction again.

Sometimes we do general induction before manipulation to prepare the area. Because of the contractility of the support tissues of the urogenital organs, induction is

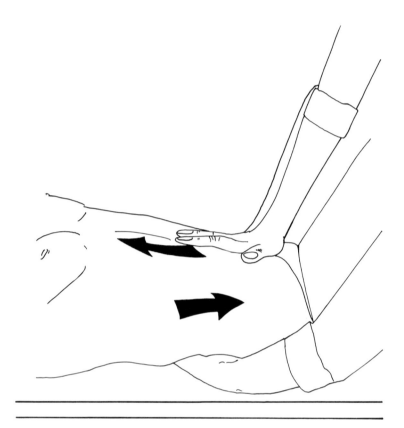

**Illustration 3-60**
Lumbogenital Induction

very important. The intrapelvic ligamentous structures are erectile; these include the vesical base, uterosacral ligaments, cardinal ligaments (lower parts of the broad ligament), and perivaginal tissues. Induction improves local tonicity by stimulating the associated muscular fibers, which also act like sponges, by helping to regulate fluid absorption and release.

## *Effects of Manipulation*

Our experiments using radiography have repeatedly shown that effective osteopathic manipulation typically restores normal mobility of restricted organs or supporting structures, and only rarely causes a change in position. Even when we have eliminated or greatly reduced pain symptoms, radiography shows no change in organ position. We conclude that *pain is caused not by improper position of an organ, but by its restriction.*

We have totally or significantly reduced pain symptoms in over 60% of cases we have treated with manipulation. The difference between radiographic and clinical results comes from the fact that the structures rediscover their mobility rather than their position. This fact brings about numerous reactions from the organism. When mobility is restored, a retroverted uterus becomes functional again, even if its position remains unchanged. We urge osteopaths, when speaking to conventional medical practitioners, to emphasize restoration of mobility rather than position!

We would like to summarize the local and general effects of manipulation.

## LOCAL EFFECTS

These are relatively specific and easy to define:
- release adhesions and restore a certain degree of elasticity to tissues;
- restore normal physiology of organs;
- improve mobility and sliding of organs;
- promote fluid circulation (arterial, venous, lymphatic, and local);
- free mechanical constraints on nerve fibers;
- reinforce tonus of perineal sphincters;
- restore normal motility and stimulate contractile structures;
- exert a local nervous reflex effect on tubular peristalsis;
- reinforce local muscular tonus;
- free osteoarticular joints;
- ease pelvic pain;
- normalize local glandular secretions.

## GENERAL EFFECTS

Since these are less specific, they are more difficult to document. In the past, when kymographic insufflation was performed to test for patency of the uterine tubes, patients would often feel a right scapular pain secondary to irritation of the subdiaphragmatic fibers of the phrenic center. During manipulation, some patients report pain at this same point. We regard this as evidence for the general effect of our manipulations.

With the use of Doppler flowmetry, we were able to show that suppression of the radial pulse, in the Adson-Wright position, could sometimes be removed by peritoneal or urogenital manipulation. We believe that this is based on a common phrenic reflex. The phrenic nerve sends a branch to the subclavicular artery which, when stimulated, is presumably capable of freeing a vascular spasm.

Who would have thought that the absence of a radial pulse with the arm abducted and externally rotated—usually attributed to subclavian artery compression—could be corrected by simply stretching the peritoneum? We knew about this phenomenon long ago because we could feel the return of the pulse under our fingers, but it became much easier to convince others once we worked out a mechanism to explain it.

Our experience leads us to believe that urogenital manipulation has a wide variety of consequences. We believe it can effect:

- the hypothalamic-pituitary axis;
- immunological system;
- endorphin production.

# Associated Restrictions

As an osteopath, you must always test the mobility of all the skeletal joints, finding any restrictions which may exist. It may be difficult or impossible to say which is the "primary" restriction; in fact, it may be of no interest to do so. Based on our experience, the following osteoarticular restrictions are most often associated with urogenital problems:

- T12/L1;
- L5/sacral or sacrococcygeal;
- right occipito-temporal;
- proximal and distal tibiofibular joints;
- navicular.

Check the joints of the feet very carefully. With urogenital problems, there is almost always an associated foot restriction which you need to manipulate.

## REFLEXOGENIC ZONES

Some of these zones are the same as those of the bladder; others more specific to the uterus:

- inguinal ligament;
- external orifice of the inguinal canal;
- attachments between pyramidalis and rectus abdominis muscles;
- pubic tubercle;
- patellar retinaculum;
- navicular and fifth metatarsal.

You will probably find others which work for you. Share your findings with your colleagues. These zones should be worked on by the classical pressure-rubbing maneuvers as first done on Chapman's reflexes.

# Precautions and Advice

Have an I.U.D. removed if you have reason to believe it will interfere with treatment or cause tissue damage. Be sure to explain your reasons to the patient. If you do this yourself it is absolutely necessary to obtain her informed consent.

Do not manipulate a pregnant patient. If there is some uncertainty (e.g., late period), postpone the appointment or modify your approach.

Arrange for the patient to come the week following her period. Even before ovulation, the estrogens cause increased tonus of the myometrium, increased frequency of contractions, and increased interstitial fluid, which increases the weight of the uterus. In the week following the period, the mucosa is flat, muscle tension is reduced, and spasms are rare. After each session, verify that there is no abnormal discharge.

Have the patient practice lying in the Trendelenburg position at home, even when there is no problem of a ptosis. This should be done with an empty stomach, lying on the ground, the pelvis resting on a stuffed chair and the legs on the chair's back. The exercise should be accompanied by breathing with ample diaphragmatic movement. Postmenopausal vascular problems are a contraindication to this exercise.

Ask the patient to carry out exercises to tonify the perineum and sphincters (described earlier) several times a day.

Warm hip baths may be helpful in cases of pelvic congestion and pain.

# Chapter Four:
## The Ovaries and Uterine Tubes

# Table of Contents

# The Ovaries and Uterine Tubes

F unctionally, the ovaries and uterine tubes (also known as Fallopian tubes) are closely related to the uterus. We are covering them in a separate chapter partly for convenience, and partly to emphasize the greater subtlety required for their manipulation. These structures require considerable precision and delicacy for both diagnosis and treatment. We are not talking about pure mechanics, but something more on the level of a craftsman's skill. We would like to start with some supplementary information on anatomy and physiology that will make it easier to understand our approach to these structures. As always, we restrict ourselves in this section to basics along with some features of these structures not noted in most books.

## Anatomy and Physiology: Ovary

The ovaries are smaller than most people think. Each ovary is approximately the size of an almond (approximately 3.5cm long, 2cm wide, 1cm thick), and weighs only 6-8 grams!

### POSITION AND CONNECTIONS

In terms of surface anatomy, the ovary is usually found on a line joining the A.S.I.S. to the superior edge of the symphysis, medial and inferior to the medial edge of the psoas.

The ovary is similar to the kidney in that osteopathic manipulation affects not so much the position or function of the organ itself, but rather the surrounding tissues (*Illustration 4-1*). When there are injuries to the peritoneum or other neighboring tissues, the ovary can become sensitive, painful, and congested. This affects its relationship with the infundibulum and fimbriae. Manipulation directly affects mobility of the ovary and kidney, and indirectly leads to such physiological effects as increased diuresis, decreased

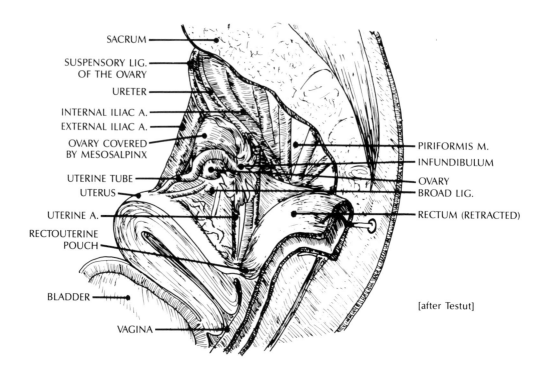

SACRUM
SUSPENSORY LIG. OF THE OVARY
URETER
INTERNAL ILIAC A.
EXTERNAL ILIAC A.
OVARY COVERED BY MESOSALPINX
UTERINE TUBE
UTERUS
UTERINE A.
RECTOUTERINE POUCH
BLADDER
VAGINA

PIRIFORMIS M.
INFUNDIBULUM
OVARY
BROAD LIG.
RECTUM (RETRACTED)

[after Testut]

**Illustration 4-1**
Ovary and its Surroundings (Posterolateral Angle)

swelling of the tissues, reduced lumbar and pelvic pain, and general improvement in the patient's condition. Important connections of the ovary are those with the:

- pelvic cavity
- infundibulum and its fimbriae
- mesosalpinx and peritoneum
- pelvic vascular system.

Position of the ovary depends on the patient's age and activities, and can often be linked to symptomatology. Most commonly, the ovary is found in the retrouterine cavity, behind the broad ligament, where it is fixed by a short peritoneal fold called the posterior wing. The ovary is posteroinferior to the uterine tube and anterior to the rectum. It is not covered by the visceral peritoneum and is free in the pelvic cavity. It is supported by several ligaments *(Illustration 4-2)*:

- the proper ovarian ligament (also known as the utero-ovarian ligament or simply the ovarian ligament) joins it to the uterine horn;
- the suspensory ligament of the ovary (also known as the lumbo-ovarian ligament) attaches it to the pelvic wall and lumbar aponeuroses;
- the mesovarium (also known as the tubo-ovarian ligament) connects the superior pole of the ovary to the outer fimbriated end of the infundibulum of the uterine tube.

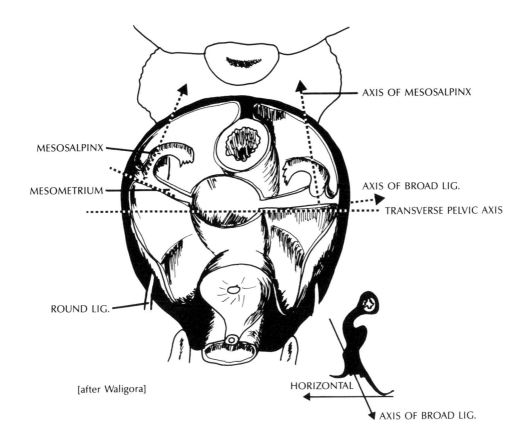

**Illustration 4-2**
Ovary: Position and Connections

The positional effect of these ligaments is debatable. We believe that the role of the suspensory ligament of the ovary is more for orientation than positioning. Some writers describe it only as a vessel-carrying fold, even though it has contractile properties. Factors such as age, sedentary life-style, and pregnancy may cause the ovary to descend farther into the retrouterine cavity or even the rectouterine pouch.

## Position of Ovary in Relation to Parity

In the nullipara, the ovary lies in the ovarian fossa, found at the bifurcation of the primary iliac artery in the lateral pelvis. This fossa represents a flattening of the peritoneal layer. In this position, the ovary lies close to the obturator nerve. This could explain certain types of knee pain in adolescent girls (described below).

In the multipara or elderly woman, as mentioned above, the ovary descends gradually into the retrouterine cavity or even rectouterine pouch. This pouch is connected to the ovarian fossa, found on the upper edge of the piriformis muscle and near its nerve (a branch of the sciatic nerve). This phenomenon explains certain types of sciatica associated with pelvic problems, as discussed below.

## Differences Between the Two Ovaries

Problems of the right ovary are often related to the cecum and appendix. The anatomical proximity and connections between these organs make differential diagnosis between them sometimes difficult. With certain problems of the cecum (particularly those caused by poor diet or malposition), the ovary may become inflamed.

Problems of the left ovary are more often related to the reproductive system. We believe that this is explained by lymphatic and venous distribution patterns and the position of the cervix (often fixed posteriorly and to the left). In a sexually active woman, such cervical restrictions often provoke pain and congestion of the left ovary. Compared to the right ovary, the left one is more affected by internal hemorrhoids.

To put it in overly simplistic and picturesque terms, one could say about the ovaries (in analogy to the kidneys) that the right one is more "digestive" while the left one is more "genital."

## Ovary and Peritoneum

We have talked to many gynecologists, obstetricians, and radiologists about the relationship between the ovary and peritoneum. Their descriptions were fairly consistent (*Illustration 4-3*). The ovary is completely intraperitoneal and is not covered by the peritoneum (i.e., lies bare in the abdominal cavity). In conjunction with the parietal peritoneum, it forms a pouch. The peritoneum is attached to the anterior edge of the

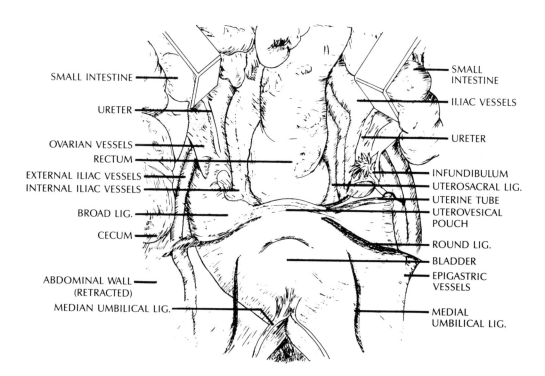

**Illustration 4-3**
Ovary and Peritoneum

ovary but stops at the boundary of the hilus (also known as Farre's white line), where it is continued by the ovarian epithelium. The posterior edge of the ovary is free. This explains why the ovary is visible and accessible during a peritoneoscopy. In earlier times, anatomists believed that two-thirds of the surface area of the ovary was peritonized, but modern methods of investigation have proven otherwise.

The mesosalpinx is the part of the broad ligament which goes from the uterine tube to the ovary and is made up of the adjoining posterior and anterior layers of the peritoneum. The posterior face of the broad ligament has a connection with the fimbriae and infundibulum which, together with the mesosalpinx, form a hood which covers the ovary.

When the uterine tube and mesosalpinx are straightened out, the ovary is not visible. Because of the intimate relationship between the ovary and peritoneum, any surgical, traumatic, or infectious damage to the peritoneum will adversely affect normal tubo-ovarian physiology. Thus, you should know how to unpleat and unfold the tubo-ovarian area.

### Obturator Nerve

This nerve crosses over the lateral face of the ovary near its superior pole, and can easily be irritated by malpositional problems of the ovary *(Illustration 4-4)*. In young women and nulliparas, the ovary may press directly on the nerve.

## MOBILITY

The ovary moves in the same way as a door on its hinges, thanks to the mesovarium and the suspensory ligament of the ovary. Its mobility depends on general, mechanical, digestive, and hormonal factors. Note that the ovary follows uterine mobility, and it is often difficult to distinguish between the movements of these two organs.

GENERAL: General factors such as age, multiparity, dystocia, sedentary life-style, and traumas can affect both the mobility and position of the ovary.

MECHANICAL: The posterior part of the broad ligament allows movement from bottom to top. The suspensory ligament of the ovary joins the ovary to the lateral wall of the lesser pelvis and subperitoneal lumbar fascia. All the other ligaments attach to mobile structures, particularly the uterus. Even the suspensory ligament of the ovary is dependent on uterine mobility as it arises from the lateral edge of the broad ligament, between its mobile and immobile parts. For example, during intercourse, the uterus moves upward in the pelvic cavity, bringing the uterine tube and part of the ovary with it.

HORMONAL: The mobility of the ovary varies with stage of the menstrual cycle. There are also hormonal variations related to emotional state, age, disease, etc.

### Other Movements

The ovary moves in response to action of the diaphragm, with pushing or retention efforts of the pelvic muscles, and during intercourse. After menopause, it swings posteriorly in the pelvis. Depending on stage of the menstrual cycle, the ovary moves closer to or farther from the uterus. Some people believe that this is due solely to the hormonal dependence of the myometrium (i.e., simple transfer of interstitial fluid in the

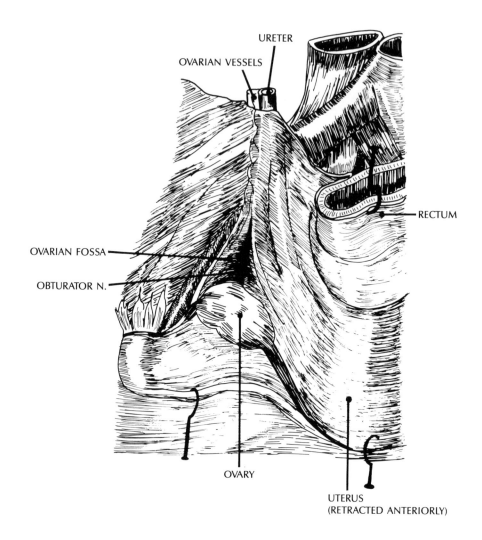

**Illustration 4-4**
Ovary and Obturator Nerve

myometrium under action of estrogens increases the weight of the uterus, which moves downward into the pelvis, giving the impression that the ovaries move upward). Others believe that the tubo-ovarian mass has its own movements, and that the ovary turns on its own axis. The latter view seems most reasonable to us. In any case, there is no doubt that some degree of motion does exist and that the ovaries and uterine tubes need to retain their proper motility in order to function normally.

## *Anatomy and Physiology: Uterine Tube*

Each uterine tube is a cylindrical duct approximately 12cm long, with a tubular canal having a width of 0.1-1.0mm at the uterine ostium and 5-7mm at the level of the ampulla. It ends with the funnel-shaped infundibulum of the oviduct, which has 12 to 14 fimbriae around the periphery, and is located close to or touching the lateral side of the ovary. The uterine tube has four radial layers (mucosal, muscular, subserosal, and serosal), and can be divided into three longitudinal parts (isthmus, ampulla, infundibulum) *(Illustration 4-5)*.

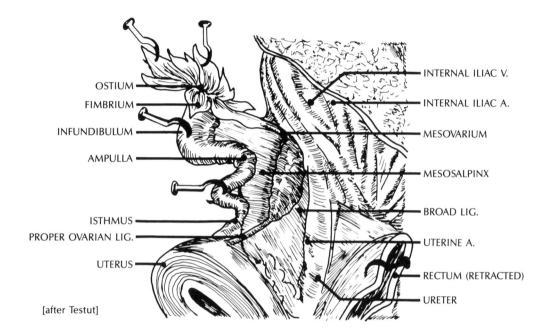

OSTIUM

FIMBRIUM

INFUNDIBULUM

AMPULLA

ISTHMUS

PROPER OVARIAN LIG.

UTERUS

[after Testut]

INTERNAL ILIAC V.

INTERNAL ILIAC A.

MESOVARIUM

MESOSALPINX

BROAD LIG.

UTERINE A.

RECTUM (RETRACTED)

URETER

**Illustration 4-5**
Uterine Tube (Posterolateral Angle)

ISTHMUS:  This is 3-6cm long and 0.2-0.4mm in diameter. It has a thick muscular layer and rich adrenergic innervation (sympathetic postganglionic fibers).

AMPULLA:  This continues the isthmus and is 5-8cm long. Its lumen becomes progressively wider distally.

INFUNDIBULUM AND FIMBRIAE:  This area measures 2-3cm in length and is lengthened by 12-14 "fringes" (the fimbriae). The abdominal ostium (see below) opens from the bottom part.

The fimbriae literally sweep the surface of the ovary. On the inside of the fimbriae and ampulla are longitudinal folds which become less distinct toward the isthmus. These are covered with secretory and ciliated cells which tend to sweep in the direction of the uterine ostium. The muscular layer and serosa are covered by peritoneal mesothelium.

## POSITION AND CONNECTIONS

The uterine tube is located in the superior wing of the broad ligament, between the ovary posteriorly and the round ligament anteriorly *(Illustration 4-6)*. Medially it is related to the small intestine, bladder, and rectum (when full). Laterally it is related to the iliac vessels, ureter, small intestine, sigmoid, and sometimes the rectum.

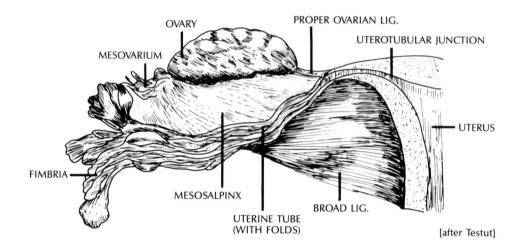

**Illustration 4-6**
Uterine Tube: Connections

## Abdominal Ostium

This is a 2-3mm wide orifice found on the lateral terminal side of the tube. It connects the pelvic region to the abdominal peritoneal region. Sperm sometimes cross over it. During a hysterography one can easily see the contrast liquid going into the peritoneum. This proves that intraperitoneal pressure is often lower than intrapelvic pressure, and that the pelvic organs tend to be pulled toward the diaphragm across the peritoneum and its contents. As far as we know, there have been no studies on the physiological role of the abdominal ostium. We believe that it may help regulate the pressure and currents of intratubal liquid, and also that our manipulations can affect the ostium by mobilizing the peritoneum and some of its attachments. Abdominal surgery, particularly appendectomy, can have a negative effect on peritoneal reciprocal forces of tension, and thus on the abdominal ostium. Such a small opening needs an environment with good distensibility.

This ostium, in conjunction with abdominal aspiration, may help account for the negative pressure observed in the uterine tubes.

## Uterotubal Junction

The lumen at this point is only 0.1-1.0mm wide. The junction is surrounded by three muscular layers going in different directions (longitudinal being predominant), and is considered to have three primary roles.

SPHINCTER-LIKE ROLE: The uterotubal junction can function like a sphincter in response to mechanical, neurological, or hormonal stimuli even though no actual sphincter has been found in this area. As osteopaths, we appreciate such sphincter-like areas (e.g., pylorus, sphincter of Oddi, duodenojejunal junction), which react well to our manipulations, often leading to a release.

SELECTIVE ROLE: The uterotubal junction functions as a "sperm trap," reducing the chance of polyspermy. For various reasons, only about 1% of the ejaculate during intercourse enters the uterus, and much less into the uterine tube itself.

ACCELERATING ROLE: During an ovulatory period, sperm can be found in the uterine tubes as little as 5 minutes after ejaculation. It is not the intrinsic speed of the sperm (12cm per hour) which explains this rapidity. We think that there is uterine and uterotubal activity which accelerates the migration of the sperm. The uterotubal junction appears to open very quickly and filter the sperm. We believe that it may even accelerate their migration.

## TUBAL LIQUID

The tubal liquid originates from both plasmatic transudation and secretion. Secretion is highest during ovulation. Tubal liquid feeds and safeguards the sperm. We believe that tubal liquid may be composed partly of peritoneal liquid, of which there is a large quantity (~ 50ml) in the abdomen. Perhaps there is also a secretory peak of peritoneal liquid around ovulation.

Interestingly, the abdominal ostium is the only example in the body of a passage between two serous cavities. There is no direct passage from the skull to the thorax, nor from the thorax to the abdomen. In hysterosalpingograms, we can clearly see the contrast liquid moving from the uterus into the tubes and finally into the abdomen. We believe the abdominal ostium and tubal liquid have significant physiological roles.

### Liquid Circulation

There exists a suction current in the pelvic peritoneum, although conversely one can sometimes find numerous particles in the uterine tubes which are present in the pelvis. In effect, during a hysterography the abdominal ostium sucks in the contrast liquid. After intercourse the sperm, aided by its own motility and this liquid current, moves toward the ovary.

Movement of the ovum in the uterine tube requires ciliary motion and the liquid current which, at this time, moves toward the uterus. Does the liquid current, at certain times and under the influence of mechanical or hormonal factors, change its direction? Fertilization normally takes place in the ampulla, and the tubal liquid appears to be indispensable for transport of the fertilized egg. Our observations suggest that the liquid current requires good condition of both uterine tubes, since one nonfunctional tube disturbs the physiological motility of the other. Similar to many other situations in the body, the reciprocal tension between the tubes must be balanced.

During the luteal phase, pressure of the liquid current is lower, but more liquid is mobilized because of uterine atony. The fertilized egg should remain 4-5 days in the uterine tube. It is held in the proximal part of the ampulla for 2-3 days because of blockage at the level of the ampulla-isthmic junction, perhaps resulting from contraction of the isthmus walls and closing of the lumen.

We have talked to many physiologists and gynecologists about this issue, and heard many points of view. At this point, we would say that good tubo-ovarian physiology requires that:

- there exists a liquid intratubal current;
- the cilia are moving;
- the uterine tubes communicate with the peritoneum (a single tubal spasm is enough to disturb tubal circulation);
- the ovary and uterine tubes are mobile;
- neurohormonal adjustments are correct.

## PHYSIOLOGY OF THE UTERINE TUBE

The physiology of the uterine tubes is complex and far from completely understood. We refer you to standard texts for an in-depth look at this fascinating and important subject. Here we will supplement that knowledge with some particularly pertinent, if somewhat simplified, information *(Illustration 4-7)*.

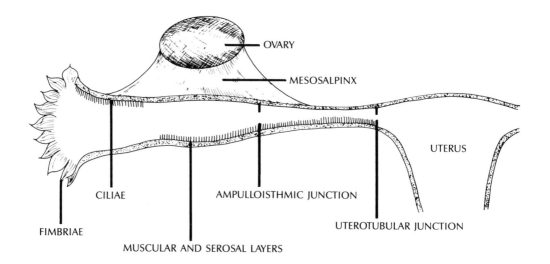

**Illustration 4-7**
Uterine Tube: Physiology

The mature ovum is released by the ovary, travels along the uterine tube, and may be fertilized by the sperm. Capture of the ovum is the major function of the infundibulum of the oviduct, whose fimbriae sweep over the ovarian surface during the ovulation phase. The smooth fibers of the ovarian ligament and suspensory ligament of the ovary, and the fibers in the very slack mesosalpinx, contract periodically in order to orient the uterine tube in a pouch-like position around the ovary. With movement, the fimbriae reach the area where the ripe follicle bursts. Ciliary movement within the tube directs the ovum toward the abdominal ostium.

As already mentioned, the sperm requires other factors besides its intrinsic means of propulsion to go so quickly toward and into the uterine tubes. Also involved in this process are the uterus, uterotubal junction, uterine tubes, and the secretory current which runs toward the ampulla. In this section we will focus on the necessary mechanical conditions for fertilization.

## Capture and Migration of the Ovum

This part of the fertilization process is dependent on several conditions:

GOOD TUBO-OVARIAN CONNECTIONS: This requires proper position of the fimbriae and infundibulum in relation to the ovary. We believe that osteopathy can help improve tubo-ovarian connections in the case of adhesions or poor elasticity of the tissues.

GOOD TUBO-OVARIAN MOBILITY: The fimbriae need to be in contact with the ovary. The infundibulum moves and the fimbriae brush over the surface of the ovary thanks to the smooth fibers of the mesosalpinx and the mesovarium. Any adhesion or lack of distensibility of these tissues will adversely affect these movements. In contrast to the infundibulum and fimbriae, the ampulla and isthmus are relatively immobile. However, they must be free of hindrances for normal function.

GOOD CILIARY MOVEMENT: The cilia of the infundibulum and ampulla tend to propel the ovum in the direction of the isthmus and uterine ostium.

OPENING OF THE ABDOMINAL OSTIUM: Proper migration of the ovum seems to depend on opening of the abdominal ostium. The current of peritoneal liquid, which (theoretically) also goes in the direction of the uterine ostium, is re-absorbed through the lumbar lymphatic nodes. Logically, one would expect that at the time of migration of the sperm, the current of the tubal liquid should either stop or be reversed. On the other hand, at the time of capture of the ovum, this current should be re-established to allow migration of the ovum. This is one of the least-understood aspects of the physiology of fertilization.

NEGATIVE INTRATUBAL PRESSURE: The pressure within the uterine tube is negative in part because of tubal contractile activity. Also important is the abdominopelvic pressure differential, particularly at the level of the abdominal ostium.

AMPULLO-ISTHMIC JUNCTION: This junction plays an important role. It tends to slow down the ovum and allow the sperm to interact with it. Fertilization, which takes place in the ampulla, must happen rapidly because an unfertilized ovum lives for only 24 hours. Once the ovum is fertilized, the ampullo-isthmic junction opens after 72 hours. These 72 hours allow the endometrium time to get ready for implantation. This time is critical. Any shortening of the 72 hour period can cause degeneration of the ovule. Any lengthening can lead to an ectopic pregnancy.

SPHINCTER-LIKE ROLE: The ampullo-isthmic junction is not an anatomical sphincter in the strictest sense. However, it has sphincter-like properties because of contraction of the muscular layer and edema of the serosal and subserosal layers.

TUBAL TRANSIT OF OVUM: Under the influence of progesterone (among other factors), the ampullo-isthmic junction opens and tubal transit of the ovum takes place via three mechanisms:

- lessening of contractile activity;
- lessening of tubal secretion;
- increase of ciliary movement.

Obviously, mechanical restraints can interfere with normal transit of the ovum.

# *Indications for Treatment*

We always have the feeling that our sections on indications are either too inclusive or grossly insufficient. It is a broad subject and it is difficult to find one's bearings. As usual, we will restrict our comments to those problems that we have actually seen in our daily practice.

## LOCAL MECHANICAL PROBLEMS

### Etiology

Causes of local mechanical problems typically fall into one of the following categories.

SURGICAL: Any surgery, particularly of the abdominal or pelvic area, inevitably affects visceral dynamics, mobility, and distensibility of tissues.

INFECTIOUS: A tubo-ovarian infection, even when treated, usually leads to adhesions and reduced tubo-ovarian mobility. In particular, sexually-transmitted diseases are very likely to negatively affect tubal transport and fertility.

TRAUMATIC: Either direct trauma to the urogenital area (e.g., in a car accident) or indirect trauma (e.g., a fall on the coccyx or a pelvic fracture) can cause tubo-ovarian problems.

OBSTETRICAL: Deliveries which are complex or too rapid often contribute to the deterioration of tubo-ovarian mechanics. We have frequently seen sequelae of ectopic pregnancies interfere with normal tubal physiology by altering the anatomical relationships between the tubes, ovaries, and surrounding tissues.

CONGENITAL: We sometimes see congenital malposition of the ovaries or abnormal flexure of the uterine tubes.

REFLEXIVE: We believe (but without conclusive evidence) that distant vertebral mechanical restrictions can trigger tubo-ovarian problems. The uterine tubes or their openings may go into spasm and disturb normal tubal physiology. Closing of the tubal lumen by spasm can be shown by hysterosalpingograms. The relationship of the sacrococcygeal area of the spinal column to the urogenital organs is well-known. With general reflexes, a distant visceral restriction can affect the tubo-ovarian axis. The most common that we have seen involves the kidneys.

Emotional factors can also contribute to tubo-ovarian problems, particularly tubal spasms. Simply calming an anxious patient during a hysterosalpingogram can release tubal spasms and improve the diffusion of contrast liquid.

## Pathology

How can mechanical pathologies disturb tubo-ovarian physiology? Remember that the uterine tube has a narrow lumen and is made up of muscular, serosal and subserosal layers with cilia which sweep in the direction of the uterus. Peristalsis is capable of somewhat enlarging the tubal lumen. The canal and its orifices can be affected by adhesion, stenosis, inflammation, flexure, or spasm.

ADHESION AND STENOSIS: These block the tubal lumen following infections. Scarring can also occur after surgical or obstetrical events. Blocking can be total or partial. Not surprisingly, manipulation is more likely to be effective in cases of partial blocking.

INFLAMMATION: With such a narrow canal, even slight edema of the serosal layer can obstruct satisfactory tubal transport. Edema can be of infectious, hormonal, or mechanical origin. Our techniques can affect tubal transport by suppressing mechanical irritation of the tissues near the tubes. We frequently see a similar "mechanical problem/tissue inflammation" relationship in osteopathy. Because of reflex and fluid effects, we can reduce inflammation by treating the mechanical problem. Other good examples are the stomach and cecum. Hiatal and esophageal inflammation can be reduced by releasing mechanical pressures on the hiatus and stomach.

FLEXURES: These can be congenital or secondary to adhesion. Flexures prevent satisfactory tubal mobility and transport. Tubal stretching seems to be most effective on noncongenital flexures.

SPASMS: The tubes and ovaries are dependent on the adrenergic and autonomic nervous systems. An irritative vertebral problem can produce a reflex tubal spasm. We do not have definitive proof that vertebral manipulation can release a tubal spasm. It would be necessary to carry out the manipulation and a hysterosalpingogram at the same time, with the risk of a placebo effect. However, as we mentioned earlier, some of our positive results on infertility were obtained by vertebral and sacrococcygeal manipulation, without anything having been said to the patient about a possible effect on her fertility. Manipulation of the cervix seems to have a particularly beneficial effect on the tubal lumen and fertility.

PERI-OVARIAN ADHESIONS: After surgery or infection, these adhesions cause pelvic and lumbar pain, as well as tubal problems. Adhesions of this type provoke pain in synchrony with the menstrual cycle, with pain usually being maximal during the premenstrual phase.

## LOCAL PAIN

### Pelvic Pain

This category includes any pain of the lower pelvis found with premenstrual syndromes, or malfunction of the organs. There may be congestive, fluid, nervous, spasmodic, mechanical, or psychological factors. Pain which appears only in the genital center often reflects a mechanical factor of tubo-ovarian or uterine origin, and may be due to spasmodic uterine contractions because of uterocervical malpositioning or uterotubal adhesions. Local tissue problems can bring about local vasoconstriction as well as visceral spasms, with an associated slowing down of venolymphatic flow.

## Abdominal Pain

INTESTINES: Abdominal pain usually involves the small intestine or large intestine. Psychological tension is almost always associated with intestinal spasms, making good results in the pelvic area more difficult to obtain. In this situation examination restricted to the pelvic area is obviously insufficient. Pay attention to the mesenteric root, sigmoid mesocolon, and attachments of the cecum to the peritoneum in particular.

KIDNEYS: Functional renal problems are often unrecognized because associated abdominal pains are confused with those of the intestine. Conventional medicine has few methods of determining a functional renal problem in the absence of associated urinary disorders.

The kidneys have a close relationship with the ovaries. Both structures can present with similar symptoms or type of pain. Symptoms include:

- swollen eyelids
- considerable morning thirst
- low back pain upon awakening
- coated tongue
- painful soles of the feet (particularly when just getting out of bed in the morning) and leg discomfort
- certain types of knee pain (see below).

Direct palpation, local listening tests, manual thermal diagnosis, and palpation of the lumbar triangle can reveal a renal problem. There is sometimes exquisite pain and tenderness between rib 12 and the iliac crest, near the transverse process of L3.

## PAIN IN OTHER AREAS

### Spinal Column

LOW BACK PAIN: This is usually of the well-known L4-L5/S1 sort with some special characteristics. Pain often follows the menstrual cycle, being maximal in the premenstrual phase. Hypersensitivity or pain with pressure on L2-L3 exists without the impression of a serious restriction or synostosis. Movement is always possible, in contrast to mechanical low back pain where problems of the nerve root, often together with those of the disc, make movement very painful.

SCIATICA: Whether left or right, sciatica is shown by the completed Lasègue test (see chapter 1). For example, when the Lasègue is positive at 40°, compression/inhibition of the ipsilateral pelvic ovarian zone produces immediate improvement in leg flexion. This does not happen in the case of nerve root pain from disc problems without visceral interference.

Compress the lower third of the A.S.I.S./pubic symphysis line. Inhibition consists of letting the palm of your hand move in the same direction as listening, and very slightly exaggerating the movement.

COCCYGODYNIA: Tubo-ovarian problems are often related to low back pain and sciatica, but less often lead to coccygodynia. Coccygodynia remains mysterious in terms of etiology. We have come across only a few cases where the ovaries were the cause.

## Legs

INFLAMED FEMORAL NERVE AND KNEE PAIN: We have mentioned the anatomical relationship between the ovary and femoral nerve. This relationship is variable depending on age, number of pregnancies and deliveries, etc. We have obtained good results on this type of pathology using simple tubo-ovarian manipulations. In these cases, the tubo-ovarian area sometimes seems congested and fibrosed, with a very obvious difference in distensibility between the two sides. Even if the mechanical problem is secondary to inflammatory and infectious factors, it still needs treatment.

Some kinds of leg pain go as far down as the lower leg. Pain of tubo-ovarian origin should never extend past the ankle joint. The cutaneous tibial ramus circulates particularly in the internal calf, and irritation of this nerve can be confused with sciatica. The internal saphenous nerve (a branch of the femoral) has a posterior terminal branch in the leg which is related to the internal saphenous vein. Its irritation also produces symptoms similar to sciatica. One of its anterior branches goes as far as the foot, and anastomoses there with a branch of the sciatic nerve, making differential diagnosis even more difficult. In this case, Lasègue sign is often absent.

## Arms

We were surprised when we first observed beneficial effects on glenohumeral pains by urogenital manipulation. The connection is not obvious. The peritoneum may be the link. Gynecologists are familiar with scapular pain set off by culdoscopy or even by insertion of an I.U.D. The lower part of the peritoneum is innervated by the lumbar and hypogastric plexuses, which in turn connect with the solar plexus. In the case of urogenital irritation, the hypogastric plexus induces pain to the solar plexus and phrenic nerves, which in turn may irritate some branches of the brachial plexus, causing cervicobrachial neuralgia.

Although we are not entirely convinced about this specific pathological process, we have no doubt that there is some nervous connection between the urogenital system and the arms. In the genitohumeral test (see chapter 1), the mobility of the glenohumeral articulation can be instantly improved by over 30% simply by mobilizing the cervix or tubo-ovarian pressure/inhibition.

Pain related to uterine or tubo-ovarian problems is mostly glenohumeral, like that of periarthritis of the shoulder. Pain rarely radiates past the lower forearm, but a painful point is often found on the deltoid-humeral attachment. Pain of this type does not have the shooting and exquisite characteristic of pain caused by cervicobrachial neuralgia of radicular origin, which can radiate as far as the fingers.

## FUNCTIONAL DISORDERS

Distinction between local and systemic functional disorders of the tubo-ovarian system is often difficult. It is likewise hard to distinguish between local functional problems and local painful problems, as they are closely interrelated. This is the case for dysmenorrhea, appearing 3-4 days before menstruation and disappearing before the end. Notable symptoms include:

- painful menstruation
- tension in the lower abdomen

- constipation
- pelvic heaviness or pain
- inguinal and femoral (anteromedial part) paresthesia
- abdominal swelling
- edema of the connective tissues
- slight knee pain.

Sometimes these local dysfunctions do not seem to be in rhythm with the menstrual cycle.

Systemic dysfunctions are often imprecise or difficult to describe. Those we have most frequently observed include:

- dysmenorrhea or amenorrhea
- weight gain
- cyclic edema
- mastodynia
- psychological problems.

A well-known example is the personality changes sometimes seen in premenstrual syndrome. These include hyperanxiety, irritability, asthenia, and depression.

## INFERTILITY

As we have said repeatedly, you must be very cautious in dealing with this subject, and avoid giving patients false hope. Every time that a couple comes to us about infertility, we talk more about our failures than our successes. Nonetheless, we are encouraged by the cases in which our techniques have helped increase fertility.

The most helpful techniques seem to be those that improve local tubo-ovarian physiology. We think our local techniques also affect regional and central nervous systems in positive ways. Stenoses, flexures, adhesions, and lack of elasticity of the uterine tubes can all be improved by our hands.

## ENDOMETRIOSIS

Some diseases are absolute contraindications for manipulation, but others, such as endometriosis, can be improved by our techniques. Even without altering the disease process, one can alleviate some of its effects. In the case of endometriosis, we cannot prevent the proliferation of endometrial tissue, but we can act upon the adhesions and accompanying spasms and pain.

# *Differential Diagnosis*

## OVARIAN CYST

The most common sign of an ovarian cyst is the presence of a mass which is independent from the uterus. These masses are painless and fairly mobile with palpation. Their movement is independent of uterine movement, which distinguishes them from fibromas (see chapter 3). Cysts can provoke dysmenorrhea or amenorrhea, with other general signs such as pallor and fatigue. There can also be compressive signs such as dysuria, constipation, and digestive disorders. You should attempt internal manipulation only after a thorough medical evaluation has been performed.

## Pedicle Torsion of an Ovarian Cyst

Patients with this condition feel sudden acute pain. They exhibit pallor, rapid pulse, nausea, vomiting, sweating, and obvious asthenia. We have never seen patients with such serious and acute symptoms as in these cases. On the other hand, we have also seen two cases of minor pedicle torsion who came to us for acute low back pain, abdominopelvic pain, and a generalized sensation of heaviness. Be alert for slight and progressive pedicle torsion, which gives symptoms of irregular, tolerable pain interspersed by periods of calm.

Intraperitoneal rupture of ovarian cysts, ovarian abscesses, or pyosalpinx (collection of pus in an oviduct) can also cause sudden acute pain, and may be accompanied by acute low back pain.

# ECTOPIC PREGNANCY

We have seen five cases of pregnancy in a uterine tube. Each of these patients consulted us for acute low back pain, and none had a history of trauma. Each came very close to an emergency situation. The case history of one of these patients is summarized below.

The patient came with her husband very early one morning, complaining of acute low back pain. We had seen her for acute low back pain many times before. This time, we were surprised to notice several unusual symptoms:

- tired appearance
- shallow, fast respiration
- facial pallor
- very sharp lumbar pain without a noticeable restriction in spinal mobility
- rapid, weak pulse
- systolic arterial pressure at 90mmHg
- lack of explanation for the low back pain.

We immediately told the husband about the possibility of an ectopic pregnancy, but he completely refused to consider this, and reminded us of the many times his wife had suffered from low back pain previously. Against his wishes, we called the emergency medical service. The patient was transported to the nearest hospital and operated on immediately, as her arterial pressure by this time was below 50mmHg.

This patient subsequently recovered and told us that she had been to see her general practitioner just before consulting us. That physician said that when he saw her she had low back pain but, at the time, the general signs of an ectopic pregnancy were slight or absent. For example, her systolic pressure was 105mmHg, a perfectly normal figure for a fairly hypotensive person early in the morning. As more symptoms appeared, the diagnosis became more obvious. We should note that early on there was no sign of peritonitis.

# PAIN IN SYNCHRONY WITH THE MENSTRUAL CYCLE

There are many possible causes of cyclical pain. The most common ovarian related ones include:

- ovarian dystrophia, characterized by acute unilateral ovulatory pain;
- dystrophic oophoritis, with the most intense pain between days 11 and 18 of the cycle;

- extremely painful cystic ovaries;
- peri-ovarian adhesions, consequences of infection or surgery which cause low back pain in synchrony with the menstrual cycle. There may be associated sciatica or leg pain which is calmed by compression or inhibition of the ipsilateral ovary (going in the same direction as local listening). Manipulation is usually quite helpful in these cases.

Another fairly common cause of this type of pain is endometriosis. It usually causes late secondary dysmenorrhea during the 2nd or 3rd day of menstruation.

## SCIATICA

Without denying that sciatica can exist because of disc disease, we find it difficult to accept every radiological diagnosis (X-ray, CT, MRI) which confirms, without doubt, sciatica due to a herniated disc. A large herniated disc may be documented by a CT scan, and yet give few or no symptoms. Conversely, we often see people with intensely painful sciatica who have little or no disc disease.

In women, a relationship between sciatica and the urogenital system is common. Characteristic signs include:

- pain in rhythm with the menstrual cycle;
- increase of pain in the premenstrual phase;
- a variable Lasègue sign depending on phase of cycle;
- signs of abdominal heaviness or pain;
- paradoxical sciatica, sometimes accompanied by paresthesia of the thigh;
- hemorrhoid crises in synchrony with sciatica and menstrual cycle;
- a positive completed Lasègue sign (improvement through pressure/inhibition on the appropriate urogenital area).

We believe that in cases of atypical sciatica, radicular pain is due to some problem with the periradicular venous system. Venous stasis of the epidural (rachidian) veins could, because of contiguity of the foramen, compress and irritate the sciatic nerve roots.

# *Demonstrating the Effects of Osteopathy*

It is very difficult to produce definitive "proof" of the effectiveness of our techniques, even though we have been actively researching urogenital manipulation for over twenty years. We have had some success in using hysterography with fluoroscopy to follow the movement of contrast liquid. When we applied direct and indirect stretching techniques at a tubal and cervical level, performed in the right direction and on the right axis, the contrast liquid moved more rapidly toward the uterine tubes and peritoneum. The same techniques, performed in a physiologically "wrong" direction, slowed down or even stopped the tubal movement. "Placebo techniques" had no effect on the movement. Similarly, in cases where transport was blocked by tubal spasm, the contrast liquid began diffusing after tubo-ovarian induction. Skeptics point out that a spasm can release itself. However, in this case, transit was notably increased at each inspir phase of the motility cycle. Again, placebo techniques had no effect. Improvement of transit occurred only when induction was correctly performed in the proper place and direction.

We have had good results as reflected by reduction of symptoms, but what really happens to the cells and tissues at which our manipulations are directed? Patients say to us, "What does it matter, since we get relief from you?" However, scientists say, "Without proof it is not real medicine." We have searched for this elusive "proof" by many means—fluoroscopy, ultrasound, CT scans, MRI, and our own manual thermal diagnosis. We have been able to document to our own satisfaction our effects on certain digestive and renal zones. But this research has usually been done privately, or unofficially in a hospital, and thus is of no use in persuading skeptics.

Infertility is a complex phenomenon, and we must be very cautious in interpreting our results in treating it. Hysterosalpingograms have revealed improvement of tubal transport following our manipulations in some cases. In other cases, though, our results have been disappointing. Before discussing some early cases which steered us toward urogenital manipulation, we would like to briefly mention the three classical effects of osteopathy.

## MECHANICAL EFFECTS

Osteopathy, in our opinion, is best known for its mechanical effects, which in turn produce the nervous and fluid effects. The osteopath's hand analyzes the condition of the tissues and determines their normality and any defects of elasticity or distensibility. If there is some problem, the fingers will try, by direct or indirect pressure, to restore proper mobility to the affected structures. For the tubo-ovarian system the fingers work on the peritoneum, ligaments (which often have contractile fibers), fasciae, and uterine tubes.

Loss of distensibility by the peritoneum disrupts good anatomical relationships between the fimbriae and infundibulum on the one hand, and the ovary on the other. A peritoneal problem can also affect the abdominal ostium by reducing abdominopelvic exchange. This exchange concerns pressure variations as well as fluids. We believe that negative intratubal pressure is due in part to the abdominal ostium, since pressure in the abdominal space is lower than that of the lower pelvis.

We believe (though without firm proof) that we can obtain release of certain spasms which are due to the contractility of lower pelvic ligaments such as the suspensory ligament of the ovary (also known as the lumbo-ovarian ligament) and mesovarium (or tubo-ovarian ligament), and that release of these spasms in turn affects tubal spasm and pelvic vasomotor response. Tubal stretching certainly influences tubal permeability through its antispasmodic effect.

## NERVOUS AND NEUROHORMONAL EFFECTS

We believe we can free various local spasms and contractions indirectly, by engaging the tissues which surround the nerves, or, in certain circumstances, the nerves themselves. It is usually impossible to differentiate between the urogenital nerves and surrounding structures, except in cases of serious neuralgia or neuritis. Local manipulations are interactive. Freeing the cervix has an effect on tubal spasms, and vice versa, as we have seen by hysterography.

It seems that all local tubo-ovarian manipulations have a general effect on the body. In fact, we believe that all local manipulations have effects on the hypothalamic/pituitary axis. But how can this be proven? We have improved some cases of amenorrhea by simply using local internal manipulations where we did not find serious restrictions.

Lansac and Lecomte (1981) postulate that when mechanoreceptors of the myometrium and cervical isthmus (which have their own contractile activity cycle) fire, they free prostaglandins which act upon smooth muscle fibers. These stimuli follow the route of visceral and perivascular sensory nerves, particularly those of the pelvic sympathetic plexus (i.e., hypogastric plexus). These sensory nerves travel up the spinal cord and reach brain centers with variable integration at the level of the cortex (intelligent vigilance), rhinencephalon (affective vigilance), and hypothalamus (vegetative vigilance). This explains the psychological, neurovegetative, and hormonal reactions to the original stimuli.

## FLUID EFFECTS

We use the word "fluid" to include veins, arteries, lymphatic vessels, and also extracellular fluids and local secretions. Some of the results of our manipulations on this fluid system can be seen with the naked eye. These include decongestion of local edema, a less bluish color of the veins, and better circulation in the lower limbs.

## CASE HISTORIES

A 35 year-old nulliparous midwife consulted us for persistent, debilitating low back pain. Osteoarticular examination showed no particular restrictions. On the other hand, all mobility and listening tests suggested a urogenital problem. We manipulated the cervix, which was fixed posteriorly, and some left lateral uterine adhesions. Six weeks later we received an irate telephone call from the patient. Her low back pain had improved, but she was pregnant! She did not want children, and had long considered herself sterile; for the past ten years she had used no contraceptive method. This is the first case that really made us believe in the efficacy of urogenital manipulations, since there was obviously no placebo effect.

Another interesting case involved the reaction of the husband of a patient, when she became pregnant after tubo-ovarian manipulation. His reaction was symbolic of the battle which exists between intellect and the facts. This man was not present at the first appointment, but accompanied his wife for the second. He seemed agitated and very nervous, almost hostile. He asked, "Was it you who, two months ago, manipulated my wife by an internal approach?" I said yes, while wondering about the reason for his agitation. "Then I have a problem," he continued. "My training as an engineer forces me to believe in coherent arguments. For the last seven years we have been from specialist to specialist, we have carried out a multitude of examinations which have sometimes been embarrassing, spent a fortune, and the slightest manipulation carried out under your care meant that my wife could become pregnant—and she is pregnant!" This engineer was caught between his own sense of logic and empirical fact. We later saw the child, who was healthy and normal.

# *Restrictions*

Certain abdominopelvic scars, because of their effect on the peritoneum and reciprocal membranous/visceral tension, disturb tubo-ovarian mobility. Uterine twisting or scarring may diminish or close the peritoneal ostium, and thereby interfere with suc-tion and tubal fluid pushing and pumping.

Adhesions and scars can occur on either the broad ligaments or their posterior wings, decreasing and disturbing the motion of the ovary in the pelvic cavity.

Restrictions of the uterine tubes and ovaries press these organs against each other, particularly in cases of sequelae and salpingitis. This can block the fimbriae or even collapse the canal.

Sexually transmitted diseases can easily lead to tubal adhesions and possible infertility. When you observe any sign of an infection, always order appropriate lab studies and a visit to a gynecologist.

Abortions or ectopic pregnancy often also lead to tubal adhesions. Don't forget to ask about these during the history.

Reflex spasms can be triggered by local or general factors, even emotions. For exam-ple, during a hysterography the anxiety of a patient can prevent the passage of the contrast liquid, i.e., the fear of not being fertile can actually prevent a patient from being so. Some reflex spasms are of hormonal origin; the uterine tubes contain hormonal receptors.

Certain local reflexes are provoked by stimulation of the peripheral nervous fibers resulting from scar tissue, and others by vertebral restrictions. Some of our results in treating infertility seem to involve these phenomena.

Finally, reduction or loss of motility in the tubo-ovarian system can affect pelvic circulation and fertility.

# *Diagnosis*

## PALPATION OF THE OVARY

The ovary is small and weighs only 6-8 grams. Palpation requires a bimanual approach; an abdominal approach by itself is inadequate. To test mobility, push the area where the ovary is located away from the vagina with the abdominal hand. Evaluate the distensibility and sensitivity of the tissues. Strong pain induced by palpation is not nor-mal. For beginners, comparison of both sides allows diagnosis of restrictions. As you gain experience, you will be able to find a restriction by exploring one side.

With your abdominal hand, compress the abdomen at the level of the mid A.S.I.S./ pubic symphysis line. Once you find the medial edge of the psoas, use two intravaginal fingers to push the lateral pouch toward the same side as the ovary that is being examined. Move the abdominal hand in the direction of the pubic symphysis while the internal fingers move superolaterally. You can usually perceive the ovary toward the lateral aspect of the pelvis. It should be only slightly sensitive; hypersensitivity is abnormal. Be extremely gentle. It is difficult to feel the ovary with any great precision. In cases of tubo-ovarian problems, the lateral pouches are often full and hard to appreciate.

## MOBILITY TESTS

### External

Place the patient in lateral decubitus position with legs bent. Explore the struc-tures on the side that is toward the table *(Illustration 4-8)*. Move from the A.S.I.S. toward the pubic symphysis, pressing posteriorly against the ilium. When the hand can move no

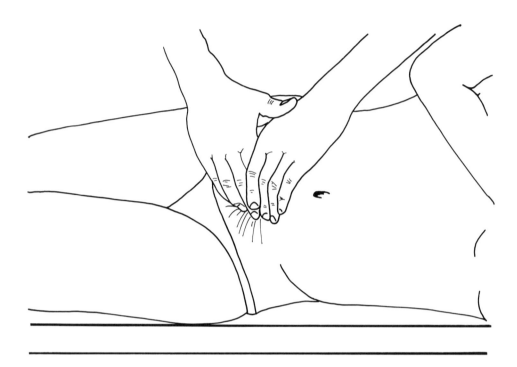

**Illustration 4-8**
Mobility Test: External

more posteriorly, direct it toward the symphysis. Evaluate tissue elasticity and note any zones of adhesion, always comparing one side with the other. If you are not sure where exactly to put your fingers, ask the patient to periodically contract the psoas, which provides a good reference point. This test can also be carried out in the modified Trendelenburg position.

### Internal

For an internal mobility test of the ovary with the patient in supine position, place two fingers in the vagina and the other hand on the abdomen. Position the abdominal hand between the A.S.I.S. and superior aspect of the symphysis and you should feel the psoas. The ovary is medial and below it *(Illustration 4-9)*. Move the vaginal hand toward the top of the lateral pouch, seeking the ovary. The two hands work together and make the tissues slide upon each other, using a back-and-forth movement of very slight amplitude. If there is a restriction, the fingers feel a granulation and diminished distensibility of the tissues. This test allows you to evaluate the broad ligament, ovary, and suspensory ligament of the ovary. These structures cannot really be differentiated from each other.

### MOTILITY TEST

With the patient in supine position, place the palm of your hand between the A.S.I.S. and symphysis, the fingers directed superolaterally. During inspir, you should feel your

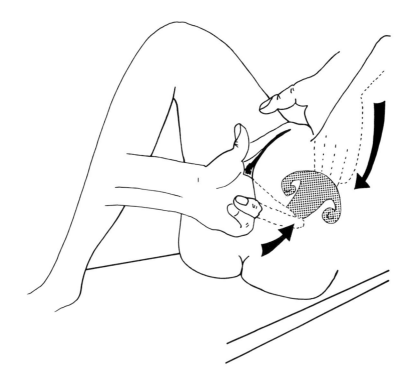

**Illustration 4-9**
Mobility Test: Internal

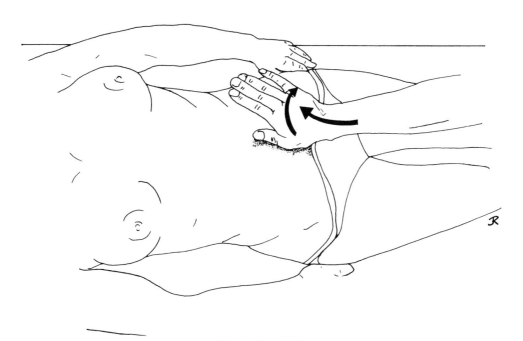

**Illustration 4-10**
Motility Test: Inspir

palm rotating laterally and slightly superiorly *(Illustration 4-10)*. That is, the left ovary seems to turn in a clockwise direction, the right counterclockwise. Once you can feel this motion easily, you will also be able to feel the lateral edge of your hand move slightly posteriorly. Presence of a restriction may diminish or abolish the movement, or even alter its direction. As always, a restriction attracts the hand. When your hand reaches the restricted zone, palpate carefully to find the exact site of injury. A motility test may enable you to discover restrictions not revealed by the mobility tests. For even greater precision, combine motility testing with local listening.

## LOCAL LISTENING

In chapter 1 we described local listening with the hand on the abdomen. Internal local listening is also possible. To listen to the uterine tubes and ovaries internally, place two fingers in the vagina, immobilize the lateral pouch on the side you want to test, and do local listening. If there is a tubo-ovarian problem, the fingers will move toward the affected area. Internal local listening reveals zones of poor distensibility which may not be found by mobility tests.

## POSITION

If there is a restriction which causes irritation near the ovaries and lateral part of the broad ligament, the patient tends to keep her legs in lateral rotation with the spine kyphosed. This position is a response to irritation of the psoas and iliac fascia, which are traversed by the iliohypogastric, ilioinguinal, femoral cutaneous, genitofemoral, obturator, and femoral nerves. Also, the subperitoneal iliolumbar connective tissue communicates with connective tissue of the broad ligaments, which leads to interdependence between the psoas and pelvis.

## *Treatment*

The purposes of tubo-ovarian manipulation include:

- defibrose and restore elasticity of the tissues;
- unfold the fimbriae;
- release the abdominal ostia;
- improve fluid circulation;
- release tubal spasms;
- reinforce tonus within the canal by stretching the uterine tubes;
- create a local/central reflex;
- stimulate the hypothalamic/pituitary axis.

The best time to manipulate the tubo-ovarian area, in our experience, is about a week after the end of menstruation. Even though we have no statistics to clearly demonstrate improved results during this period, the tissues seem to react more rapidly and without irritation at this time. Manipulation is not contraindicated during other parts of the cycle, though we ourselves avoid the actual period of menstruation.

We have heard some people advise doing internal manipulations with a bare hand. This is potentially dangerous for both patient and practitioner. Always wear gloves. Make sure they are kept clean.

## EXPLANATION TO THE PATIENT

Patients may be apprehensive of the discomfort and possible pain of urogenital examination and treatment. We always take the time to carefully and professionally explain to the patient what we are going to do. As a result, none of our patients has ever refused to be treated. You should explain to the patient the following facts about internal manipulation:

THEY ARE VERY COMMON: These techniques are routinely used for such common problems as pelvic pain, low back pain, and infertility.

THEY ARE PAINLESS: Only movements which lift the cervix, where there are adhesions or partial ruptures of the uterosacral ligaments, may be slightly painful at the beginning. There are few reactions following treatment, aside from slight tensions or abdominopelvic heaviness, both of which are temporary.

THEY DO NOT TAKE LONG TO PERFORM: Urogenital tissues react very quickly to manipulation because of their great sensitivity and the quick reactivity of contractile fibers (ligaments). Precise and rapid techniques are essential for good results. Osteopathic principles demand that we give information to the body in order to provoke a good reaction. Overly prolonged techniques tend to make the messages locally received by the body relatively trivial, and prevent autocorrective reactions. Ten minutes of internal work should be the maximum.

THEY REQUIRE ONLY A FEW SESSIONS: Two or three sessions should be sufficient to obtain a positive result. If not, the patient should discontinue osteopathic treatment and consult other specialists. In accordance with the osteopathic principle of letting the body take care of itself, always let one menstrual cycle pass between consecutive treatment sessions. Too-frequent sessions interfere with the body's autocorrective process. The best reaction is often obtained after the first session because the body is "surprised" by the new stimulus.

THEY DO NOT POSE DANGER TO THE PATIENT: Our techniques are gentle and respect the delicate urogenital system. As far as we know, we have never caused adverse iatrogenic effects either in the short, medium, or long term. Be particularly careful around an I.U.D. so that you do not destabilize it.

THEY ARE USEFUL, SOMETIMES INDISPENSABLE: A deep urogenital restriction requires internal manipulation since it cannot be affected by the external approach.

## EXTERNAL TECHNIQUES

### Mobility

External manipulation for mobility is done in the same position as the test. The patient is in the lateral decubitus position with legs bent. Stand behind the patient so you can manipulate the region nearest the table. Delicately free the restriction by stretching the tissues toward the medial side of the ilium, then toward the median uterine axis, then superiorly, and lastly, inferiorly. It is important to stretch the tissues on all planes. Remember the position of the restriction so you can work on it internally.

**Induction**

After performing either of the techniques described below, conclude with a general uterovesical induction movement.

ABDOMINAL INDUCTION: Your fingers are positioned as for listening to motility of the ovaries. If you feel no movement at all, start it up again by encouraging inspir seven or eight times during one minute. The palm of the hand rotates laterally and moves slightly superiorly, while the lateral edge of the hand presses slightly deeper. If the movement you feel is disturbed, let your hand go in the direction of the restriction, and exaggerate slightly the abnormal direction so that you may gradually rediscover the right direction.

LUMBO-OVARIAN INDUCTION: Place one hand under the lower lumbar vertebrae and the other over the ovary to be treated. While the ovary hand carries out a lateral rotation, the lumbar hand will tend to move superiorly and slightly toward the side opposite the treated ovary (Illustration 4-11). This technique seems to act on the contractile fibers of the suspensory ligament of the ovary.

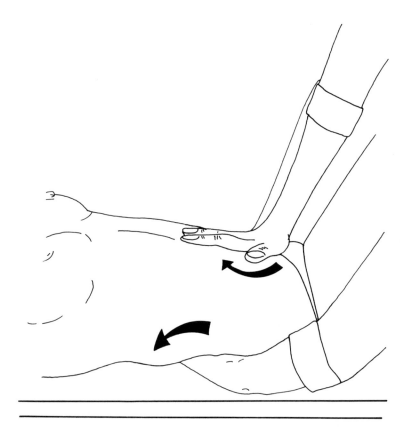

**Illustration 4-11**
Lumbo-ovarian Induction

## INTERNAL TECHNIQUES

### Stretching the Lateral Pouches

You need to free the lateral pouches before beginning actual tubo-ovarian manipulations.

DIRECT TECHNIQUE: The patient lies in supine position with hips flexed. Use two intravaginal fingers to surround the cervix and evaluate the presence and distensibility of the lateral pouches. These may be absent if the cervix is lying against the vaginal wall. In this case, try to introduce a finger between the lateral ipsilateral wall of the vagina and the cervix, playing upon both elements in turn. It is good to work upon the lateral pouches alternately at first, and only then simultaneously, separating the two lateral vaginal walls from each other. If this is unsuccessful, tackle the posterior pouch in order to move the cervix anteriorly. This technique, thanks perhaps to a reflex action provoked by stretching the uterosacral ligaments, has the beneficial effect of opening the lateral pouches.

LISTENING TECHNIQUE: After completion of direct technique, place your two fingers in the two lateral pouches, and move in the direction of listening. Treatment is finished only when local listening disappears. The aim of this technique is not to reshape the pouches, which may remain in the same condition at the end of the session as before. The goal is to activate connections between local/regional and local/central stimuli on the mechanoreceptor fibers of the lateral pouches.

### Mobilization of Ovary

This follows the same protocol as the test. The abdominal fingers move toward the ovary from the cervical region and the intravaginal fingers position themselves under the ovary. Using both hands, carefully surround the ovary and move it superolaterally away from the uterine axis. Let it return. This is repeated gently and rhythmically 4-5 times until the movement is easy to carry out. Once the ovary is mobilized, gently stretch all the zones that were found to be restricted. With a corpulent woman, you will probably be unable to clearly feel the ovary or tubes. However, with a woman of normal weight and after sufficient experience, you should be able to feel these structures well and sometimes "uncap" the lateral end of the tube from the ovary by a slight rotational movement. We must emphasize again the importance of gentleness and delicacy when manipulating the ovary. We often tell our male students to do this technique as if they were manipulating their own testicles. Believe me, they immediately become much gentler!

### Cervical Orifice Technique

This technique is often helpful for infertility. Use it only after stretching the lateral pouches. Presence of an I.U.D. or infection are contraindications.

DIRECT TECHNIQUE: First, you need to find the cervix and bring it forward. If the cervix remains in anterior position, you can work with one finger. If it will not stay anterior, use one finger to maintain its position, and the other finger to carry out the technique. The motion used is only slightly greater than that of listening.

Place your finger on the cervical orifice and push it slightly inward. Play upon the internal walls of the cervix laterally and from top to bottom. This technique should be very gentle; you are not trying to penetrate the orifice by force. You are trying to provide local stimulation to enlarge the cervical lumen and provoke a general reflex action. For fertilization to take place, the sperm must obviously be able to pass freely through the orifice. Some cervixes seem to be inhibited, and this technique stimulates them. By first freeing the lateral pouches, the cervix can be stimulated and thus become more accessible. Nevertheless, this technique can be difficult or even impossible with hypotonic cervixes.

LISTENING TECHNIQUE: The finger slightly presses in the direction of the orifice, following intracervical local listening. Gently and slowly exaggerate the movement and follow it until it stops. Usually, listening will make you first go toward the internal edges of the cervix, and then out radially toward the uterine cavity.

### Cervical-ovarian Stretching

Again, you need to stretch the lateral pouches prior to this technique. Then place one or two fingers in the ipsilateral lateral pouch, and the abdominal hand on the lower third of the A.S.I.S./symphysis line. To get in position, the abdominal hand presses medially and posteriorly in the direction of the ovary.

DIRECT TECHNIQUE: Use the internal hand to push the cervix in the direction of the contralateral pouch, while the abdominal hand moves in an inferolateral direction as if it wished to rejoin the A.S.I.S *(Illustration 4-12)*. This technique allows tubal stretching

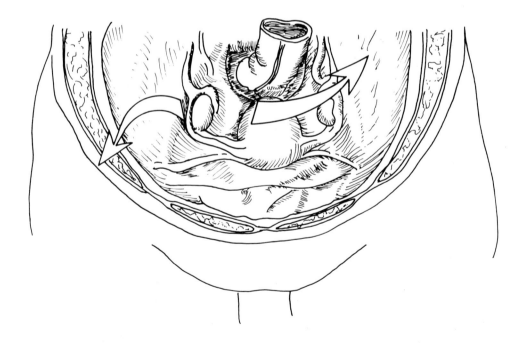

**Illustration 4-12**
Cervical-ovarian Stretching

and freeing of the peri-ovarian tissues. Do not be aggressive with the abdominal hand; this may stimulate contraction of the abdominal muscles and tube, leading to intestinal or ovarian pain.

LISTENING TECHNIQUE: Once the internal fingers (in the ipsilateral lateral pouch) exert a slight traction, they can be left to follow the direction given by listening. Simultaneously, the abdominal hand moves in the direction it feels on listening. These two directions of listening may not necessarily be the same.

## Tubo-ovarian Stretching/Unwinding

This can be performed following cervical-ovarian stretching by adding medial or lateral rotational movements of the abdominal hand. However, the following method is more precise. Move the two internal fingers superolaterally, toward the A.S.I.S., while the fingers of the abdominal hand go toward the internal fingers as if trying to meet them (Illustration 4-13). These movements should be slow and of limited amplitude. The ovary can be felt between the internal and abdominal fingers. As usual, it is not easy to differentiate the ovary (a tiny round mass) from surrounding tissues. Once you have found it, surround it with your fingers and move it laterally toward the internal face of the pelvis. Next, perform medial and lateral rotational movements to have an effect at the level of the uterine tubes, fimbriae, infundibulum, abdominal ostium, and mesovarium.

LISTENING TECHNIQUE: Tubo-ovarian stretching/unwinding should be followed by listening. After bringing the ovary toward the internal face of the pelvis, gently maintain this stretching and follow the movements indicated by listening. You will have the impression of the ovary moving over slightly-stretched elastic. These movements are minute and require considerable delicacy on your part. We consider this the "queen of techniques" for the tubo-ovarian system.

## Abdominovaginal Induction

The abdominal hand is above the ovary. This hand and the two intravaginal fingers carry out induction of the ovary together. For the left ovary, during inspir there will be a clockwise movement (frontal plane) associated with a slight anterior sliding (parasagittal plane) and lateral rotation (transverse plane). The hands return to their original position during expir. This technique need only be performed 3-4 times. We often use this as the first intravaginal technique.

# *Conclusion*

Nothing in the lower pelvis is completely fixed. All the organs and connective structures move against each other. The liver has powerful ligaments (coronary and triangular ligaments) which attach it to the relatively fixed (or at least predictable) diaphragm. Tubo-ovarian motions are more complex than those of the liver because the ovary and uterine tubes are attached to structures (e.g., uterus) which not only move, but are themselves variable in position. These combined and complex motions make evaluation and treatment difficult. Except for the uterosacral ligaments and parametria, all ligaments of the uterus, tubes, or ovaries only "fix" the organs in the vaguest sense of the word, leaving them always a subtle mobility.

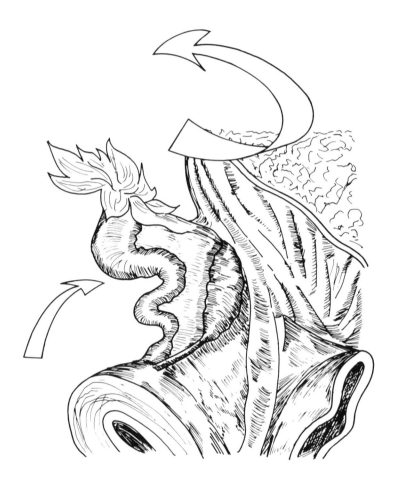

**Illustration 4-13**
Tubo-ovarian Stretching/Unwinding

The complex process of sperm meeting ovum requires optimal mobility and elasticity of structures such as the:

- fimbriae and infundibulum
- uterine tube
- uterus
- peritoneum,

and proper opening of sphincter-like regions such as the:

- abdominal ostium
- ampullo-isthmic junction
- tubo-ovarian junction
- cervix.

Without wishing to make the factors of fertilization too mechanical, we believe that it is clear that osteopaths can take pride in our ability to treat this area with our craft. Adhesions and other consequences of urogenital infections (including sexually-transmitted ones) frequently interfere with fertility, especially as these diseases become more common and difficult to treat. Osteopathic manipulation can often be successful in helping relieve the pain these problems can cause. Sometime we can even help them regain their fertility.

# Chapter Five:
## Conclusion

# *Conclusion*

To help a woman become a mother, or to free her from the stigma of incontinence—these are within the capability of the osteopath using the techniques we have presented here. Apart from practitioners of manual medicine like ourselves, who could possibly have the necessary delicacy and skill to accomplish these things? "To have such delicacy and skill"—what a wonderful expression, and what a noble aim.

## A "TYPICAL" SESSION

We are often asked what happens during a typical session. Of course, each session is different, and what we do depends on what restrictions we find, the physical condition of the patient, and so on. Always remember that preconceived ideas have no place in the osteopathic concept. We must treat whatever restrictions we find. That said, in general our best results are achieved by applying techniques in the following order:

COCCYX: An untreated restriction of the coccyx can cause treatments elsewhere to fail, or reduce the duration of their effects. A common mistake is to test the inferior end of the sacrum instead of the coccyx. Do not hesitate to put the finger evaluating coccygeal movement as far forward as necessary.

ABDOMEN: Be wary of restrictions of the intestines or omentum, which can lead to restrictions in the urogenital system. You can stretch the junction between these two regions by lifting the entire intestinal mass. Adhesions of the small intestine can affect not only the bladder, but also the uterine tubes and ovaries.

CERVIX: Cervical restrictions bring about reflex tubal spasms. To obtain good results on the uterine tubes and ovaries, you must free the cervix first.

TUBO-OVARIAN SYSTEM: The ovaries and tubes travel throughout the lesser pelvis. Disruptions in their motion can have widespread effects.

SPINAL COLUMN: We usually obtain better results by manipulating the spinal column after the viscera. Freeing visceral restrictions removes slight vertebral reflex restrictions. This prevents us from overstimulating the reflex vertebral arcs. Once the tubo-ovarian system is freed, it reacts much better to reflex stimuli induced by vertebral manipulations, particularly at the level of the sphincter-like areas. Spinal restrictions associated with those of the tubo-ovarian system are commonly found at T11, L1, L3, and sacrum. Slight painful restrictions to L3 which permit nearly-normal articular movement are often a sign of reflex genital problems (such as infection, endometriosis, fibroma, or tumor).

KIDNEYS: Problems of the left kidney tend to affect urogenital structures, and vice versa. When you encounter vascular problems of the lower pelvis, the left kidney should always be checked. Based on embryological development and our own experience, it seems that treating the left kidney affects not only the urogenital system, but also the central hormonal system. Manipulation of this kidney is useful in treating impotence in men, any local or general genital malfunction, or vascular problems of the lower pelvis.

CRANIUM: Address cranial problems only after all local restrictions have been treated. We often find posterior cranial restrictions associated with urogenital problems. Stimulation, both of the rhythm and of the amplitude, of the primary respiratory motion can also be useful for urogenital problems.

## CLOSING THOUGHTS

We have consistently tried to integrate the abilities of our hands and medical technology in order to confirm our diagnoses and refine our manipulations. Whenever possible, osteopathic medicine should use objective experimentation. This helps enhance our status in both the medical and scientific communities. We know that our skills can help people, but we must convince others of this. We must also continually strive to make our manipulations more and more precise and effective.

Therapeutic work on the female urogenital system demands great subtleness and respect for the patient. It goes further than mere technique. It requires a broad sense of compassion and teaches us to respect life in all its stages and forms. Osteopaths can help patients with urogenital problems for which the relational handicap is worse than the pain. Our ability, using external and internal manipulation, to relieve problems that might otherwise require surgery, makes us indispensable.

Use of our own fingers to restore normal function—is that not the ideal of our profession?

# Bibliography

Barral, J-P. *The Thorax.* Seattle: Eastland Press, 1991.

Barral, J-P. *Visceral Manipulation II.* Seattle: Eastland Press, 1989.

Barral, J-P., Ligner, B., et. al. *Nouvelles techniques uro-génitales.* Verlaque, 1993.

Barral, J-P., Mathieu, J-P., Mercier, P. *Diagnostic articulaire vertébral.* Charleroir: S.B.O.R.T.M., 1981.

Barral, J-P., Mercier, P. *Visceral Manipulation.* Seattle: Eastland Press, 1988.

Beck, R., Hsu, N. "Pregnancy, Childbirth and the Menopause related to the Development of Stress Incontinence," *American Journal of Obstetrics and Gynecology* 91 (1965): 820-23.

Bochuberg, C. *Traitement ostéopathique des rhinites et sinusites chroniques.* Paris: Maloine, 1986.

Braunwald, E., et. al., eds. *Harrison's Principles of Internal Medicine.* New York: McGraw-Hill, 1987.

Chaffour, P., Guillot, J-M. *Le Lien mécanique ostéopathique.* Paris: Maloine, 1985.

Comroe, J. H. *Physiologie de la respiration.* Paris: Masson, 1978.

Contamin, R.; Bernard, P., Ferrieux, J. *Gynécolgie générale.* Paris: Vigot, 1977.

Crobier, A. *"Trou obturateur" énigme ostéopathique.* unpublished thesis, 1991.

Cruveilhier, J. *Traité d'anatomie humaine.* Paris: Octave Doin, 1852.

Davenport, H. W. *Physiologie de l'appareil digestif.* Paris: Masson, 1976.

Delmas, A. *Vois et centres nerveus.* Paris: Masson, 1975.

Dousset, H. *L'examen du maalade en clientèle.* Paris: Maloine, 1972.

Drye, J.C. "Intraperitoneal Pressure in the Human," *Surgical Gynecology and Obstetrics* 87 (1948): 472-475.

Enhörning, G. "Simultaneous Recording of Intravesical and Intraurethral Pressure: A Study on Urethral Closure in Normal and Stress Incontinent Women." *Acta Chirurgia Scandinavia* (1961), suppl. 276.

Gabarel, B., Roques, M. *Les fasciae.* Paris: Maloine, 1985.

Green, T. H. "Urinary Stress Incontinence: Differential Diagnosis, Pathophysiology, and Management," *American Journal of Obstetrics and Gynecology* 122 (1975): 368-400.

Grègoire, R.; Oberlin, S. *Précis d'anatomie.* Paris: J.P. Balliére, 1973.

Huges, F. Cl. *Pathologie respiratoire.* Paris: Heures de France, 1971.

Hugier, J., et. al. "Les soutènements vésico-uretraux," *Encyclopedie Mèdico-Chirurgicale: Techniques Chirurgicales* (1968): 30-41.

Hutch, J. A. "A New Theory of the Anatomy of the Internal Urinary Sphincter and the Physiology of Micturation: The Base Plate and Micturation," *Obstetrics and Gynecology* 30 (1967): 309-17.

Issartel, L.; Issartel, M. *L'ostéopathie exactement.* Paris: Robert Laffont, 1983.

Kahle, W.; Leonhardt, H.; Platzer, W. *Anatomie des viscères.* Paris: Flammarion, 1978.

Kamina, P. *Anatomie gynécologique obstrétricale.* Paris: Maloine, 1984.

Kolodny, R.; Masters, W.; Johnson, V. *Textbook of Sexual Medicine.* Boston: Little, Brown and Company, 1979.

Korr, I. *The Neurobiologic Mechanisms in Manipulative Therapy.* NY: Plenum, 1978.

Laborit, H. *L'Inhibition de l'action: Biologie, physiologie, psychologie, sociologie.* Paris: Masson, 1981.

Lansac, J.; Lecomte, P. *Gynécologie pour le praticien.* Villeurbanne: Simep, 1981.

La Vielle, J., Roux, H., Stanoyevitch, J.F. *Le système vertébro-basiliaire.* Marseille: Sola, 1986.

Lazorthes, G. *Le système nerveux périphérique.* Paris: Masson, 1971.

Malinas, Y. and Favier, M. *A. B. C. de Mécanique obstrétircale*. Paris: Masson, 1979.

Poirier, P., Charpy, A., Nicolas, A. *Traité d'anatomie humaine*. Paris: Masson, 1912.

Prefaut, C. *L'Essentiel en physiologie respiratoire*. Paris: Sauramps Mèdical, 1986.

Raz, S., et. al. "The Vascular Component in the Production of Intraurethral Pressure," *Journal of Urology* 108 (1972): 93-6.

Renaud, R., et.al. *Les incontinences urinaires chez la femme*. Paris: Masson, 1980.

Robert, J.G., et.al. *Précis de gynécologie*. Paris: Masson, 1974.

Rouvier, H. *Anatomie humaine*. Paris: Masson, 1967.

Scali, P., Warrel, D. W. *Les prolapsus vaginaux et l'incontinence urinaires chex la femme*. Paris, Masson, 1980.

Susset, J. G., et. al. "Urodynamic Assessment of Stress Incontinence and its Therapeutic Implications," *Surgical Gynecology and Obstetrics* 122 (1976): 343-49.

Taurelle, R. *Obstétrique*. Paris: France Mèdical Edition, 1980.

Testut, L. *Traité d'anatomie humaine*. Paris: Octave Doin, 1889

Testut, L., Jacob, O. *Anatomie topographique*. Paris: Gaston Doin, 1927.

Tournaire, M., et. al. *Physiologie de la reproduction humaine*. Paris: Masson, 1985.

de Tourris, H., Henrion, R., Delecour, M. *Gynècologie et obstrètrique*. Paris: Masson, 1979.

Upledger, J. E., Vredevoogd, J. D. *Craniosacral Therapy*. Seattle: Eastland Press, 1983.

Waligora, H., Perlemuter, L. *Anatomie*. Paris: Masson, 1975.

Waligora, H., Perlemuter, L. (II) *Abdomen et petit bassin*. Paris: Masson, 1975.

West, J. B. *Physiologie respiratoire*. Paris: Medsi, 1986.

Williams, P., Warwick, R, eds. *Gray's Anatomy*. Edinburgh: Livingstone, 1980.

Wright, S. *Physilogies appliquée à la médicine*. Paris: Flammarion, 1974.

# List of Illustrations

CHAPTER THREE

## CHAPTER FOUR

# Index